PUBLIC HEALTH IN THE 21ST CENTURY

VITAMIN A AND LUNG DEVELOPMENT

PUBLIC HEALTH IN THE 21ST CENTURY

Additional books in this series can be found on Nova's website under the Series tab.

Additional E-books in this series can be found on Nova's website under the E-book tab.

NUTRITION AND DIET RESEARCH PROGRESS

Additional books in this series can be found on Nova's website under the Series tab.

Additional E-books in this series can be found on Nova's website under the E-book tab.

PUBLIC HEALTH IN THE 21ST CENTURY

VITAMIN A AND LUNG DEVELOPMENT

M. L. PINTO
P. RODRIGUES
A. HONÓRIO
C. GONÇALVES
AND
V. BAIROS

Nova Biomedical Books
New York

For permission to use material from this book please contact us:
Telephone 631-231-7269; Fax 631-231-8175
Web Site: http://www.novapublishers.com

NOTICE TO THE READER

Library of Congress Cataloging-in-Publication Data

Vitamin A and lung development / M.L. Pinto ... [et al.].
p. ; cm.
Includes bibliographical references and index.
ISBN 978-1-61761-311-1 (softcover)
1. Lungs--Growth. 2. Vitamin A--Physiological effect. I. Pinto, M. L.
[DNLM: 1. Lung--growth & development. 2. Vitamin A. WF 600]

QP121.V545 2010
612.2--dc22

2010031454

Published by Nova Science Publishers, Inc. † New York

Contents

Preface

Lung development is a methodical and coordinated process that culminates in the creation of an organ that contains airways, alveoli, and blood vessels. Lung development also has multiple innate and acquired host defense systems and processes that weaken the harmful effects of oxygen in the environment. By regulating cellular differentiation and branching morphogenesis, vitamin A, in particular, its active metabolite retinoic acid, plays an essential role during lung development. Retinoic acid is required for normal alveolar development and vitamin A administration increases lung's elastic fiber contents at birth. Additionally, several experiments showed that retinoic acid restores alveolar architecture to dexamethasone-treated lungs and maintains alveolar development in lungs treated with an angiogenic inhibitor. Clinical trials revealed that vitamin A supplements given to premature infants decreased death and respiratory disorders due to lung immaturity, such as respiratory distress syndrome and bronchopulmonary dysplasia. On the other hand, for vitamin A deficiency, the incidence for diseases of the respiratory tract is considerably increased. Throughout pregnancy, maternal mechanisms of vitamin A homeostasis are mobilized to ensure that adequate levels of retinoids are available and reach the embryo and fetuses through accurate mechanisms of transplacental transfer. Nevertheless, given the fundamental roles of retinoids in embryonic development it is of vital importance that the conceptus should form its autonomous vitamin A reserves and be capable of maintaining normal levels of this compound. The present chapter reviews original and published research on vitamin A signaling pathways during lung maturation, outlining the morphogenetic effects of this compound on the temporal and spatial expression of several molecules involved in lung organogenesis, as well as their possible variation according to sex, since an adult lung presents sexual dimorphism. The issues regarding the effects and benefits of vitamin A administration during the pre-natal periods are discussed. The storage and distribution capacity of the maternal-fetal unit in response to vitamin A supplementation during gestation are also addressed by discussing the distribution of retinol and retinyl palmitate levels in the mother's plasma, liver, lung, placenta, amniotic fluid and milk, as well as in the liver and lung of fetuses. However, vitamin A functions are not limited to the prenatal and growing periods, but are also indispensable for the maintenance of the different populations in the adult organism, namely in the lung, where the retynil palmitate levels change remarkably in response to vitamin A administration.

Chapter I

Introduction

In mammals, the moment of the first breath is crucial. The newborn should be fit for this important challenge, which occurs suddenly at birth, and for successfully establishing the alveolarization of the lung. Postnatal lung function is critically dependent upon optimal embryonic lung development. As such, the speed of the lung's maturation is of great importance for all medical conditions dealing with premature birth. The process of lung development and maturation results in the formation of an organ that contains airways, sophisticated gas exchange units (alveoli), blood vessels, multiple innate and acquired host defense systems, and mechanisms to counteract the adverse effects of oxygen in the environment. Lung development is a highly ordered and coordinated process that can be divided into five stages or periods. According to their different morphological features the stages of lung development are named embryonic, pseudoglandular, canalicular, saccular and alveolar. Depending on the mammal species, the alveolar phase can begin during late gestation, as occurs in humans, or after birth. An impairment of alveolarization has been implicated in the pathogenesis of respiratory distress syndrome (RDS) and bronchopulmonary dysplasia (BPD), a disease that affects premature newborns. Approximately 80 years ago, Wolbach and Howe (1925), described the squamous metaplasia of the conducting airway epithelium as a consequence of vitamin A deprivation. They also found out that this effect could be reversed by vitamin A repletion (Torday & Rehan, 2004). Since this first study, numerous works have supported the importance of vitamin A and its active metabolite, retinoic acid (RA) in lung morphogenesis, homeostasis, and repair. Retinoic acid seems to be the most active of the retinoids in terms of interaction with the genome. Analysis of a

RA reporter mouse model reveals that RA activity is at its highest during the initiation of lung morphogenesis (Malpel *et al.*, 2000), regulating early airway branching, structural remodeling during development leading to alveolar formation and the synthesis of surfactant (Cardoso, 2004). Therefore, it is not surprising that vitamin A deficiency during gestation causes serious abnormalities in lung development, including lung hypoplasia and lung agenesis (Shi *et al.*, 2009). Although severe vitamin A deficiency has been controlled effectively (Sommer, 2003), in some countries, mild or marginal vitamin A deficiency (MVAD) is still a serious and widespread public health problem in pregnant woman and children (Ngare *et al.*, 2000; Barón *et al.*, 2003). Clinical trials revealed that vitamin A supplementation given to premature infants had decreased death and respiratory disorders due to lung immaturity, such as respiratory distress syndrome and bronchopulmonary dysplasia.

In this chapter, research on vitamin A signaling pathways during lung maturation, as well as the advantages and caveats associated with using pre-natal and post-natal vitamin A supplementation are outlined.

Chapter II

Stages of Lung Development

Embryonic Stage

In humans during the 4th week of embryonic development, lung start to appear as a diverticulum from an outgrowth of the ventral wall of the primitive foregut. This diverticulum is lined by epithelial cells derived from the endoderm germ layer, and is covered with splanchnic mesoderm. Epithelial cells of the primitive foregut invade the surrounding mesenchyme and undergo repetitive, dichotomous branching to form the proximal structures of the tracheo-bronchial tree (Joshi & Kotecha, 2007). The branching pattern displays right/left assimetry, as lung buds initially form three diverticula in the right lung bud and two in the left that correspond to the lobes of the adult lungs. As mentioned, branching morphogenesis gives rise to the right and left primary bronchi, then the secondary (lobular) bronchi, the tertiary (segmental) bonchi and so forth (McGowan & Snyder, 2004). There is no consensus regarding the mode of development of the 6th branchial arch artery from which the pulmonary artery develops, but recent studies suggest that the pulmonary arteries and veins develop *in situ* within the splanchnic mesoderm surrounding the foregut via at least two processes that seem to occur concurrently: (a) vasculogenesis, in which new blood vessels form *in situ* from angioblasts and (b) angiogenesis, which involves sprouting of new vessels from existing ones. A third process, called fusion, is required to connect the angiogenic and vasculogenic vessels, thus expanding the vascular network (Stenmark & Abmann, 2005). Distal angiogenesis, described as the process in which the formation of new capillaries from the pre-existent ones occurs at the periphery of the lung, further ensures the coordinate expansion of a vascular network as branching proceeds (Parera *et al.*, 2005).

Pseudoglandular Stage

During the pesudoglandular stage of lung development, which in humans lasts from 6 to 16 weeks of gestation, repeated branching of the bronchial tree continues (Figure 1A) (Cardoso & Lu, 2006), in a process that results in more than 10^5 conducting airways. Later in lung development, remodeling of the bronchial tree will give rise to more than 10^7 respiratory airways arrayed in an intricate pattern crucial for oxygen flow (Mauroy *et al.*, 2004).

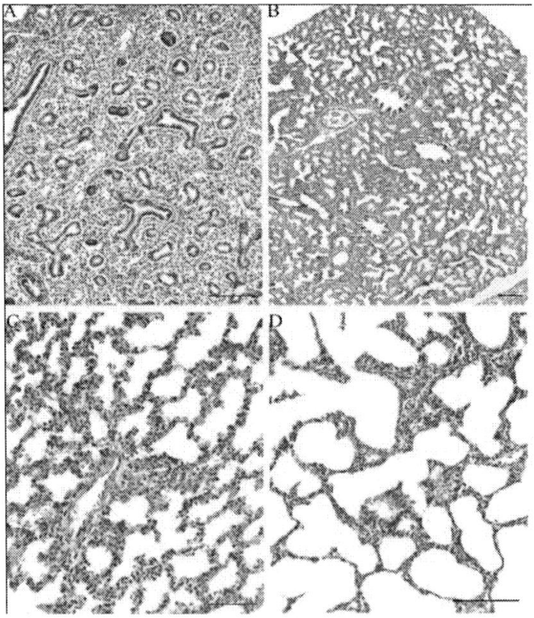

Figure 1. Histological features of the different stages of lung development in mice. During the pseudoglandular stage (A-15 gestational days) repeated branching of the bronchial tree occurs. The canalicular stage (B-17 gestational days) is characterized by remodeling of the distal portion of the branching duct system and proliferation of the capillary network. At the saccular stage (C-18 gestational days) further branching of the terminal portions of the duct system takes place, which gives rise to the alveolar sacs. In the alveolar stage (D-day of birth) protusion of secondary crests from the primary septa leads to the formation of primitive alveoli. H-E; Scale bars: A, B and D=100μm; C=50μm.

Pattern of airway branching and division is determined by epithelial–mesenchymal interactions. Bronchial mesenchyme induces branching in the trachea, whereas tracheal mesenchyme inhibits branching of the bronchial tree (Warburton *et al.*, 2000; Cardoso & Lu, 2006). In advance gestation the process of differentiation follows a centrifugal pattern: maturation begins in proximal (large) airways and spreads distally. At the end of the pseudoglandular stage, mesenchyme has already begun to differentiate into cartilage and bronchial smooth muscle.

This phenomenon is accompanied by epithelial differentiation, which gives rise to the ciliated cells, mucous and serous cells, basal cells, Clara cells and neuroendocrine cells, among other phenotypes in the proximal airways. Sumucosal glands are already noticeable at the late pseudoglandular stage of lung development (Jefferey, 1998).

During this phase, the epithelial cells lining the distal portions of the conducting airways remain undifferentiated as tall columnar cells with large pools of intracellular glycogen (McGowen & Snyder, 2004). Despite of this, the first molecular marker of distal epithelial differentiation expression, the surfactant protein gene SP-C is detected in the mouse lung in about 10.5 gestational days, when secondary buds form (Wert *et al.*, 1993).

Canalicular Stage

During the 16th to the 24th weeks of gestation in humans, remodeling of the distal portion of the branching duct system to form the respiratory bronchioles and alveolar ducts occurs (Figure 1B). The canalicular stage of lung development is also characterized by the proliferation of the capillary network around the terminal ducts (Joshi & Kotecha, 2007). The connective tissue components of the lung derived from the splanchnic mesoderm proliferate actively (cartilage, smooth muscle, etc). Around the 20th week of gestation, some of the distal epithelial cells become more cuboidal and present multilamellar bodies in the cytoplasm. This indicates their differentiation into alveolar type II cells, which begin to synthesize and release surfactant. At the same time, capillaries in the interstiticium induce the overlying epithelial cells to flatten and differentiate into alveolar type I cells (McGowan & Snyder, 2004).

Saccular Stage

This phase of lung development, which in humans takes place between the 24 weeks of gestation and the onset of birth, is marked by the lengthen, dilation, and further branching of the terminal portions of the duct system, giving rise to the alveolar sacs (Figure 1C). This ensures increased surface area for gas exchange. During this stage, there is also further differentiation of type II cells to type I cells and increment in surfactant production. In humans, it is estimated that 15-18% of true alveoli form late in gestation, however the bulk are formed after birth (McGowan & Snyder, 2004).

Alveolar Stage

Alveolar formation is recognized by the septation of the alveolar sacs. This process is termed secondary septation and is initiated by the protusion of secondary crests from the primary septa (Figure 1D), which are the walls of the alveolar sacs. The secondary crests are in close relationship with elastic fibers and arise where the capillaries in the primary septum can be folded up, giving rise to a double capillary layer. The increase in the height of secondary septae is accompanied by an increase in the number of multilamellar bodies and surfactant production. The subsequent remodeling of this alveolar wall is characterized by the further lengthening and thinning of secondary septae, primarily via the loss of interstitial mesenchymal cells and extensive capillary remodeling. The original dual capillary system gradually becomes a single capillary system in which the capillaries are interconnected trough a process named intussusceptive microvascular growth (Buri *et al.*, 2006). Alveolar multiplication continues in the postnatal period at least up to the age of 2-3 years and alveolar size and surface increases until after adolescence in humans (Kotecha, 2000; Hislop, 2002).

Chapter III

Vitamin A Signaling Pathways during the Early Stages of Lung Development

Although timing of the stages of lung growth in animals do not mimic that of human, numerous elegant animal studies on rodents have given us a better understanding of the influence of vitamin A as a key factor regulating lung growth. All-*trans* retinoic acid (RA) is the major biologically active metabolite of vitamin A, acting through the transcription factors RARs and the retinoid receptors RXRs. Both types of receptors have tree isoforms (α, β, and γ) which heterodimerize to form the functional unit that transduces RA signaling (Rodrigues *et al.*, 2004).

RARs and RXRs are expressed during lung development beginning at the earliest stages (Dollé *et al.*, 1990; Mollard *et al.*, 2000, Dollé, 2009). However, retinoic acid requirements for proper lung organogenesis start earlier in embryonic development. In fact establishment of endodermal cell fate and foregut morphogenesis are dependent on the correct temporal and spatial expression of numerous transcription factors, including *Gata 4*, reported as regulated by RA (Arceci *et al.*, 1993; Doi *et al.*, 2009). Subsequently, the spatial expression of these transcription factors and several other molecules along the anterior-posterior axis of the gut endoderm defines organ-specific domains, as occurs in the region that will become the lung primordium. In mammals, signaling between Fgf10 (fibroblast growth factor 10) in the mesenchyme and Fgfr2 (fibroblast growth factor receptor 2) expressed by the endodermal epithelial cells is crucial for lung bud morphogenesis (Bellusci *et al.*, 1997; Park *et al.*, 1998). This pathway illustrates the constant cross-talk between the endodermal-derived lung bud and the surrounding mesenchyme during in all stages of lung development. It has been shown that *Fgf10* expression and bud formation in the lung field is critically dependent on RA (Desai *et al.*, 2004). After an increase on RA synthesis and use detected throughout the gestational days 8.5-9.5 in mouse foregut (Malpel *et al.*, 2000), lung primordial buds form at gestational day 9.5. In the presence of an RA antagonist, explants of foregut cultured at gestational day 8.5 fail to form lung buds through *Fgf10* signaling (Desai *et al.*, 2004), a mechanism that seems to be mediated by RARβ in the mesoderm (Desai *et al.*, 2006).

Left-right differences in pattern are first recognized when secondary buds form, and continue to develop as branching morphogenesis proceeds, which results in lung assymmetry, with more lobes in the right lung (4 in the mouse and 3 in humans) than in the left (1 in the mouse and 2 in humans) (Cardoso, 2001). Lung asymmetry is determined by several factors, including Tgfb-related (transforming growth factor beta) molecules, such as activin receptor 2, *Lefty1*, *Lefty2* and growth differentiation factor 1, *nodal* (Lowe *et al.*, 2001), and by the bicoid type homeobox gene *Pitx2* (Cardoso & Lu, 2006). Studies with mice whole-embryo cultures revealed that RA is necessary for expression of some of these genes, including *Lefty*, *nodal*, and *Pitx2* (Chazaud *et al.*, 1999), therefore implying its capacity to directly influence left-right lung asymmetry and branching.

Retinoic acid signaling during the early stages of lung development is further reinforced with studies that show that as it happens with disruption of RA signaling in the foregut (Mollard *et al.*, 2000), deletion of *RARα* and *RARβ* (Mendelsohn *et al.*, 1994), as well as deletion of either *Fgf10* or *Fgfr2* in mice (Sekine *et al.*, 1999; De Moerlooze *et al.*, 2000) leads to lung agenesis and multiple abnormalities. Interestingly, lung phenotypes exhibited by mice with *RAR* and *RXR* gene deletions are similar, albeit more complex, to those observed in the fetal and postnatal VAD (vitamin A deficiency) syndromes (Mark *et al.*, 2006). Also, no lungs are formed in mice deficient in the RA-synthesizing enzyme RALDH2 (retinaldehyde dehydrogenase) (Desai *et al.*, 2004; Wang *et al.*, 2006).

The subsequent branching morphogenesis that results in the formation of the bronchial tree in mice takes place between gestational days 10.5-17, and occurs at sites where branching is stereotypically determined by *Fgf10* expression. The precise location of *Fgf10* expression is dynamic, since it appears to precede distal bud formation, being down-regulated once the bud is formed (Bellusci *et al.*, 1997). One of the major inhibitors of *Fgf10* expression in the mesenchyme is the growth factor Tgfβ1, which also inhibits epithelial cell proliferation and differentiation (Serra *et al.*, 1995). Furthermore, Tgfβ1 induces synthesis of extracellular matrix, what seems to prevent local branching when deposited in the epithelial mesenchymal interface (Heine *et al.*, 1990). Interestingly, it is the endogenous RA that controls Tgfβ activity in the prospective lung field to allow local expression of Fgf10 and induction of lung buds (Chen *et al.*, 2007). Secondary branching, however, is characterized by a marked down-regulation of RA signaling in lung epithelia and mesenchyme (Malpel *et al.*, 2000). This was previously demonstrated by studies that showed that treating lung organ cultures with RA disrupts distal lung formation and maintains the lung in a proximal-like stage (Cardoso *et al.*, 1995, 1996). These effects result partially from decreased RA synthesis, but also from increased RA degradation in the epithelium via P450RAI-mediated metabolism, and inhibition of RA signaling in the mesenchyme by COUPTF-II expression. In the distal regions of these lungs the expression and distribution patterns of Fgf10 and Bmp4 (Bone morphogenetic protein-4), which is a member of the Tgfβ superfamily of growth factors normally expressed at high levels at the bud tip epithelium, are altered (Malpel *et al.*, 2000). The former studies illustrate the importance of regional mechanisms that control RA availability and utilization for the correct expression of genes that are essential for distal lung formation, thus illustrating the complexity of RA effects during lung morphogenesis.

Chapter IV

Vitamin A Signaling Pathways during Lung Maturation

The effect of vitamin A and its active metabolite-RA on lung development is balanced by the interplay between RA and its receptor subtypes. During lung branching morphogenesis, *Rarβ* remains expressed along the endoderm of the trachea and the proximal (large) bronchi, but is absent in the distal bronchi and the developing alveolar epithelia, while *Rarγ* is expressed in a more homogeneous manner in developing lung tissues (Dollé *et al.*, 1990). In fact, at the pseudoglandular stage, RA signaling through RARβ, but not RARγ, inhibits distal bud formation thereby promoting the formation of conducting airways. Furthermore, it appears that the level of CRBPI (Cellular retinol binding protein I) in the pseudoglandular lung also participates in the control of branching morphogenesis (Mollard *et al.*, 2000). As mentioned before, epithelial cells derived from the endoderm in the branching ducts undergo cellular differentiation, giving rise to the specialized cells that line the conducting and respiratory airways at the pseudoglandular stage of lung development. There are approximately 40 different cellular phenotypes in the lungs of adult mammals, and their differentiation seems to be the most critical process in the successful function of the lung. At least eight of these cell phenotypes line the tracheal bronchial conducting airways, including the ciliated cells, basal cells, mucous goblet cells, serous cells, Clara cells, small mucous granule cells, brush cells, neuroendocrine cells, and a number of undifferentiated or partially differentiated cells (Plopper & Fanucchi, 2004). Vitamin A is required for the preservation and induction of the expression of differentiated functions in the tracheobronchial epithelium. In primary hamster tracheal epithelial cultures vitamin A treatment enhances the proliferation of small mucous-granule cell type (McDowell *et al.*, 1987; De Luca & McDowell, 1989) while in human tracheal bronchial epithelial cells it induces the expression of at least four mucin genes. The regulation of these genes appears to be mediated by RARα and RARγ (Gray *et al.*, 2001). On the other hand, vitamin A deficiency causes keratinizing squamous metaplasia of the mucociliary epithelium, which is accompanied by a reduction in the synthesis of mucous glycoproteins. However, this process can be reversed by vitamin A or retinoid administration (Plopper & Fanucchi, 2004).

The majority of studies aimed at unraveling vitamin A effects during fetal development are performed during late gestation, at the onset of the alveolar stage, which is probably related to the teratogenic activity of this compound. Our research, however, delves into the influence of vitamin A during the time span that comprises both fetal and post-natal lung maturation. During the late pseudoglandular and canalicular stages of development, lung undergoes marked epithelial and mesenchymal differentiation, proliferation, and remodeling. Multiple signaling pathways, growth and transcription and factors, as well as several molecules regulate the previously mentioned processes in a precise temporal and spatial manner, allowing undisturbed lung morphogenesis and organogenesis. Among other factors, Fbf and vascular endothelial growth factor (VEGF) particularly, are key players during the pseudoglandular and canalicular stages of lung development (Kumar *et al.*, 2005). As its name implies, VEGF is a potent mitogen for endothelial cells, playing a fundamental role in angiogenesis and vasculognesis, but its functions are not limited to vessel development (Abman, 2003). In fact, VEGF induces a significant increase in both epithelial- and endothelial-branching morphogenesis (Del Moral *et al.*, 2006), and accelerates lung growth in rat fetal lung explants (Shinkai *et al.,* 2006). This double action upon epithelial and endothelial cells is not surprising, taken into account that recent data indicate that the formation of pulmonary vascular units directs epithelial morphogenesis (Cardoso & Lu, 2006). Moreover, vessel development in the early lung is crucial for lung structure maturation, and both undisturbed angiogenesis and vasculogenesis are necessary for the successful building of the organ (Healy *et al.,* 2000; Voelkel *et al.,* 2006), as evidenced by studies that show that inhibition of angiogenesis decreases alveolarization in the developing rat lung (Jakkula *et al.*, 2000). Importantly, VEGF altered expression is a common feature on some of the most important lung diseases: infants dying from BPD have reduced pulmonary levels of VEGF (Bhatt *et al.*, 2001), and it has been reported that there is a substantial decrease of this growth factor in an experimental model of persitent pulmonary hypertension of the newborn (Abman, 2007). Concerning the aspects that pertain to lung branching morphogenesis and vessel development, it is important to notice that RA is required to control endothelial cell maturation and cell cycle progression during vasculogenesis and angiogenesis (Lai *et al.,* 2003), and that vitamin A is one of the regulators of VEGF expression in the lung (Pinto *et al.*, 2007). One of the studies performed by our group included the morphological analysis of VEGF, regarding its expression and distribution pattern in the fetal and neonatal lung, as well as the quantification of VEGF pulmonary and plasma levels after vitamin A administration. For that, a single dose of vitamin A was injected subcutaneously to pregnant female mice at the 12th day of gestation, when lungs were at the late embryonic stage. Samples were collected daily from the 15th gestational day till the day of birth. Since the exogenous supply of vitamin A was administered at a time of gestation when in principle the well-known teratogenic effects of vitamin A are no longer to be felt, no animals at all times presented any malformations. The morphological study of lung VEGF during the different stages of lung development was performed by immunohistochemistry, while pulmonary and plasma VEGF levels were quantified by ELISA. Both methods revealed that at gestational day 15, VEGF expression in the lung of control fetuses is higher than the one observed in vitamin-A-treated fetuses (Figures 2 and 3). Lungs from control fetuses display a strong immunostaining for VEGF that can be observed in the cytoplasm of mesenchymal cells, epithelial cells of the tubular respiratory tree and in the extracellular matrix (Figure 2A and B). However, VEGF plasma levels were higher in fetuses whose mothers had received vitamin A (Figure 4).

In the canalicular stage, 16th gestational day, when angiogenesis and vasculogenesis are a prominent feature in the fetal lung, and in the remaining stages of lung development, a progressive increase of VEGF pulmonary levels (Figure 2C and D; Figure 3) and a decrease of VEGF plasma levels were observed in mice whose mothers had received vitamin A (Figure 4). On the opposite, VEGF pulmonary levels suffer variations and VEGF plasma levels showed a gradual and sustained increase throughout development in control mice. At the day of birth, VEGF pulmonary levels and immunoexpression patterns in control and vitamin A treated neonates are similar.

It seems that plasma and pulmonary VEGF change inversely, raising the hypothesis that lung could act as the physiological reservoir of this growth factor (Kaner & Crystal, 2001). Albeit lung presents the highest level of VEGF gene expression among normal tissues (Kaner *et al.,* 2000; Voelkel *et al.,*

2006), the assumption that the variations of VEGF plasma levels during fetal development would reflect VEGF variations in the developing lung needs further confirmation.

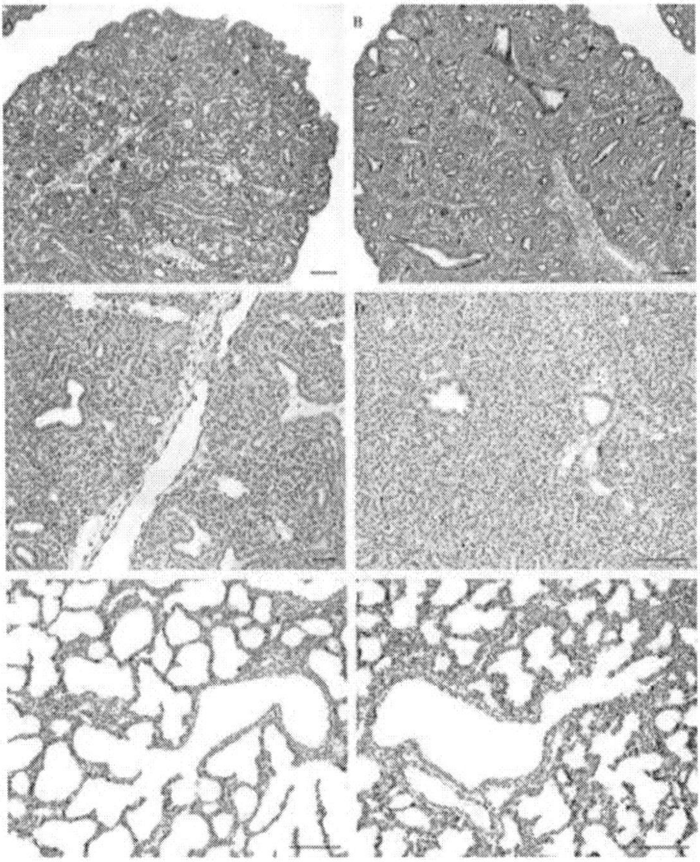

Figure 2. Immunohistochemistry for vascular endothelial growth factor (VEGF) in the lungs of mice. At the 15th gestational day (pseudoglandular stage), VEGF expression in the lung of control fetuses (A) is higher than the one observed in vitamin-A-treated fetuses (B). Inversely, at the 16th gestational day, a decrease o VEGF pulmonary immunoexpression occurs in control animals A (C), when compared to fetuses exposed to vitamin A (D). At the day of birth, VEGF immunoexpression patterns in the lung of control (E) and vitamin-A-treated (F) neonates are similar. Scale bars=100μm.

Preliminary results from our research also indicate that VEGF lung content is higher in females from the control group, especially on the critical period before birth, which suggests that during normal gestation both the angiogenic and the overall lung maturation processes are favored in female fetuses.

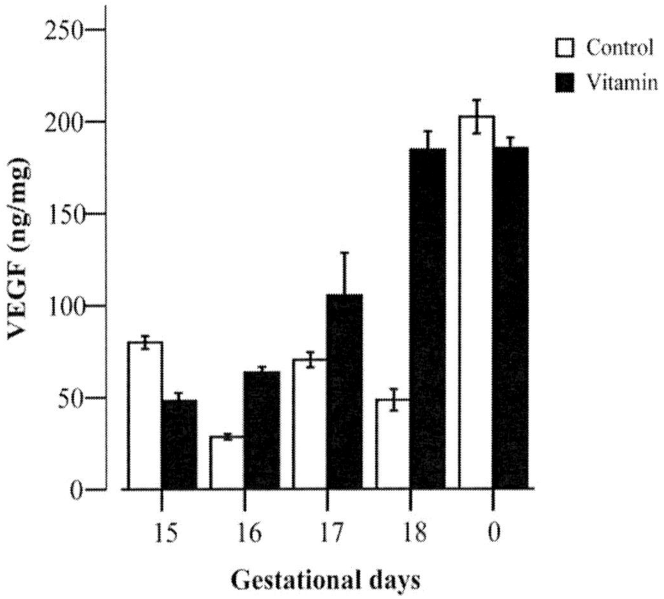

Figure 3. Vascular endothelial growth factor (VEGF) levels in the lungs of mice during fetal development and in the newborn expressed in ng of VEGF / mg of protein (mean ± SD). A gradual increase of VEGF pulmonary concentration is observed in animals exposed to vitamin A during gestation, which peak at the perinatal period. In control animals VEGF pulmonary levels ten to be lower than in vitamin-A-treated fetuses, especially at the end of gestation (18th gestational day).

It is likely that the abundance of estradiol and progesterone in the female fetus are at the origin of higher VEGF lung content, since recent studies show that the combined treatment with these hormones enhances VEGF synthesis in mice embryonic alveolar cell type II and central lung fibroblast cultures. Moreover, in alveolar cell type II cultures there is a concomitant increase of surfactant proteins SP-B and SP-C synthesis (Trotter *et al.*, 2009a).

Blocking estradiol and progesterone receptors in piglets during the end of the gestational period often decreases SP-C mRNA expression and alveolar counts. This effect is mainly due to the reduction of alveolar counts in males, which display diminished alveolarization. In newborn piglets, VEGF and surfactant protein SP-B are higher in females, but this difference is abolished when estradiol and progesterone receptors are blocked (Trotter *et al.*, 2009b). Although sexual dimorphism of the adult lung has been well established

(Massaro *et al.*, 1995, 1996; Massaro & Massaro, 2004, 2006), these findings suggest that gender differences occur earlier during lung development. This hypothesis is supported by the fact that in humans, respiratory function of very prematurely born infants is influenced by sex, being characterized by a female advantage. Male premature infants have lower body weight and require more days of oxygen therapy than females (Thomas *et al.*, 2006; Carey *et al.*, 2007). The existence of gender differences, with a female advantage, regarding surfactant synthesis during lung development is also well documented in humans and several animal models (Adamson & King, 1984; Torday, 1984; Fleisher *et al.*, 1985; McMillan *et al.*, 1989). Our research shows that maternal vitamin A administration influences fetal and neonate VEGF pulmonary and plasma levels, and that vitamin A seems to work in a synergetic manner with VEGF through their morphogenetic effects to enhance lung development, a process which will occur earlier in females.

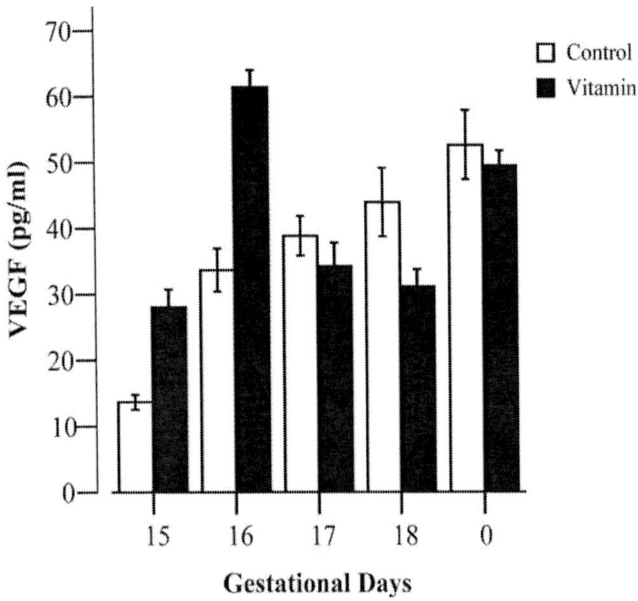

Figure 4. Vascular endothelial growth factor (VEGF) levels in the plasma of mice during fetal development and in the newborn expressed in pg of VEGF / ml (mean ± SD). A sustained increase of VEGF in the plasma of control fetuses is visible through out the gestational period. However, VEGF plasma levels are highest at the 16th gestational day in fetuses subjected to vitamin A influence. At the day of birth both control and vitamin-A-treated newborns display similar values of VEGF plasma levels.

As mentioned before, branching morphogenesis and vessel development require constant tissue remodeling, which in turn depends of dynamic epithelial-mesenchymal interactions mediated trough the coordinated expression of cell adhesion molecules, growth factors, cytokines, chemokines, and constant extracellular matrix turnover. Proteolytic cleavage of the former substrates, achieved by the highly coordinated action of matrix metalloproteinases (MMPs) and their physiological inhibitors, tissue inhibitors of matrix metalloproteinases (TIMPs), is one of the major regulators of lung tissue remodeling. By their proteolytic activity, MMPs can affect the adherence of cells to the extracellular matrix and, on the other hand, release both bioactive fragments of extracellular matrix molecules and "trapped" bioactive mediators, providing signals from the microenvironment to cells allowing them to react to stimuli (Gueders *et al.*, 2006; Greenlee *et al.*, 2007). Retinoic acid controls the expression of several members of the MMPs family at the tanscriptional level (Ludwig *et al.*, 2000; Balmer & Blomhoff, 2002). Our group performed a morphological study of the ontogeny of MMP-1 and MMP-9, as well as their tissue inhibitor TIMP-1, during the different stages of lung development in mice fetuses and neonates subjected to vitamin A influence during the gestational period. MMP-1 expression is weak or absent at the pseudoglandular stage, strong at the first day of the canalicular stage (16th gestational day), but decreases at the 17th gestational day, increasing again at the saccular stage of lung development. Although MMP-1 and MMP-9 expression patterns are different during the stages of lung development under study, prenatal administration of vitamin A modified only MMP-9 immunorreactivity (Figure 5). On the contrary, the observations revealed that TIMP-1 expression is high during all stages of fetal lung development and also in neonates. Because of its influence upon MMP-9 lung's expression, vitamin A also induces an unbalance of the MMP-9/TIMP-1 ratio. As such, the marked anti-proteolytic profile at the 16th gestational day and a proteolytic profile at the last gestational day are displayed in the lungs of fetuses exposed to vitamin A. Since MMP-9 is the main cause of the proteolytic degradation of extracellular matrix components in the basement membrane, namely type IV collagen (Atkinson & Senior, 2003, Chakrabarti & Patel, 2005), the maternal administration of vitamin A seems to promote the active remodeling of this structure, and therefore may anticipate the establishment of a functional blood-air barrier at the alveolar wall.

During the last stage of lung development, the process by which saccules transform into alveolar units involves formation of secondary septa from the pre-existent walls and represents the last major event of lung morphogenesis

(Cardoso, 2001) Alveolarization is critically dependent on vitamin A both for chemical (surfactant) and structural maturation. Vitamin A deficiency during gestation causes reduced expression of surfactant proteins SP-A, SP-B, and SP-C in fetal lung, depicting an impairment of distal epithelial differentiation (Chailley-Heu, 1999).

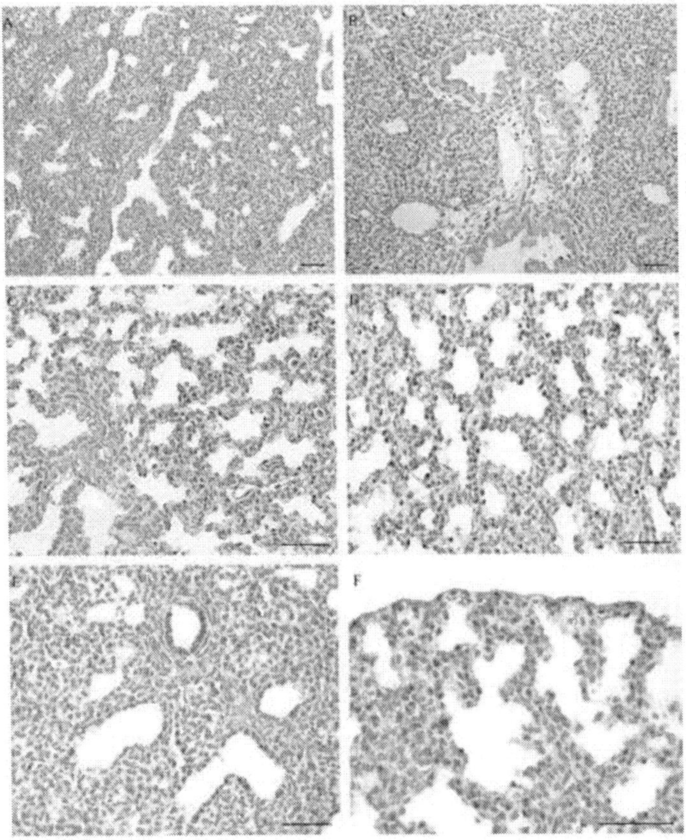

Figure 5. Immunohistochemistry for matrix metalloproteinase-9 (MMP-9) and tissue inhibitor of metalloproteinase-1 (TIMP-1) in the lungs of mice. In the lung of control fetuses MMP-9 expression is higher at the 16th gestational day (A). In vitamin-A-treated fetuses there is a decrease in MMP-9 expression at this day (B), but a progressive enhancement of its expression can be observed. At the 18th gestational day MMP-9 immunoexpression is higher in the lungs of animals developed under the influence of vitamin A (C), when compared to control animals (D). TIMP-1 expression is high during all stages of lung development (E -16th gestational day; F- 18th gestational day). Scale bars: A, B, C and D=100μm; E and F=50μm.

On the other hand, a temporal association between the appearance of bundles of elastic fibers at the tips of the secondary septa and the formation of new alveoli occurs, providing evidence that elastic fibers are one of the structures supporting the secondary septa during the alveolization period (Fukuda *et al.*, 1984). The process of elastin synthesis and deposition seems to be initiated by lipid-droplet laden pulmonary interstiticial cells, called lipofibroblasts, present at the regions undergoing secondary septa formation (Burri, 1974). Lipofibroblasts store retinoids, mainly in the form of retinyl esters (Shenai & Chytil, 1990), and synthesize elastin in response to RA (Bruce *et al.*, 1998). Coordinated with the physical process of septation, as well as the alveolar epithelial cell differentiation; stores of retinyl esters decline in the lung, implying that lipofibroblasts may release retinol locally, which in turn can be metabolized to RA in retinoid-sensitive tissues, such as the epithelial and interstitial lung components (Geevarghese & Chytil, 1994). Moreover, lipofibroblasts synthesize and secrete RA suggesting that retinoid signaling occurs in a paracrine fashion (Dirami *et al.*, 2004). The idea that RA could regulate alveolarization first came out from the study by Massaro & Massaro. (1997). It demonstrated that all-*trans* RA administration to newborn rats increased the number of alveoli, decerased their size and increased the surface area of the lungs. On the other hand, studies where the alveolarization process was disrupted by treatment either with dexamethasone (Hind & Maden 2004; Maden & Hind 2004; Maden 2006) or an angiogenesis inhibitor (Cho *et al.*, 2005), and restored afterwards trough the administration of RA, further depicted the fundamental role of this metabolite during the final stage of lung development. Studies in RAR mutant mice suggest that RA can act as a positive or a negative regulator of alveolization depending on the RAR type. RARβ-null mice septate earlier and faster than control mice, while RARγ-null have decreased alveolar number and an increase in alveolar volume, an effect that is exacerbated with the simultaneous delection of one RXRα gene (Massaro *et al.*, 2000; McGowan *et al.*, 2000).

Taken together, the results provided by the morphological and biochemical studies herein mentioned indicate that vitamin A modulates lung morphogenesis through intricate signaling pathways, which involve the regulation of VEGF, MMP, TIMP, and elastin expression. The functional relevance of the correct temporal and spatial expression of the molecules mentioned earlier is further reinforced by the fact that their expression changes under medical conditions in which lung immaturity is a common feature, such as premature birth or BPD (Bhatt *et al.*, 2001; Winkler *et al.*, 2003).

Chapter V

Biometric and Morphological Data from Lungs Developed under the Influence of Vitamin A

Body weight is one of the most important parameters to access fetal viability. Data on mice fetal weight are scarce, however a systematic approach performed during several years of studies by our group focusing on fetal development under physiological conditions allowed us to establish the normal range of fetal body weight for this species. The same approach was also used regarding lung weight during the time period that encompasses the pseudoglandular, canalicular, sacular, and the onset of the alveolar stages of mouse lung development. This enabled the assessment of the lung's relative weight (lung weight/body weight), which at the end of gestation is, on average, similar for rats (Antipatis *et al.*, 1998) and mice (3,28% and 3,83%, respectively). It is noteworthy that in mammals, lung's relative weight at the end of gestation is higher than in newborns (Schellenberg et al., 1987).

The administration of vitamin A on the 12th gestational day results in an increase of mice fetal body weight measured at 14th – 18th gestational days (Figure 6).

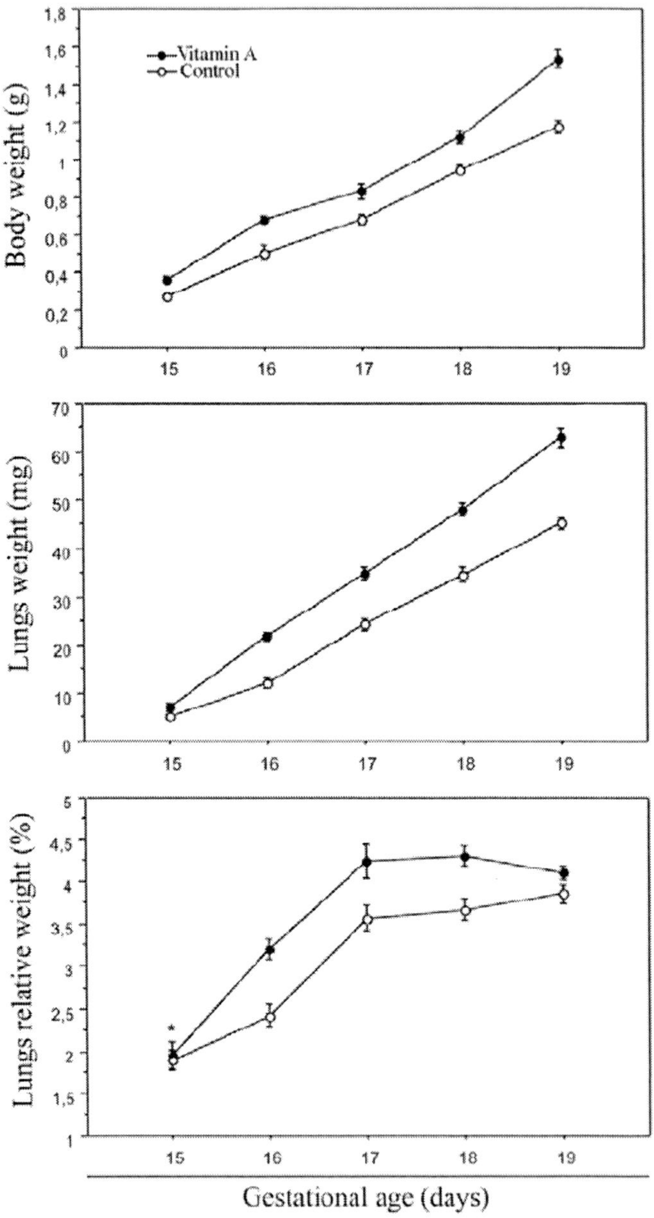

Figure 6. Body weight, lung weight, and lung's relative weigh during fetal development in mice (mean ± SD). Fetuses developed under the influence of vitamin A display higher body and lung's weight through out the gestational period.

In the last day of gestation, mice exposed to vitamin A are, on average, 1,3 times heavier than mice developed under physiological conditions. Despite reports that directly relate the increase on fetal growth with a reduction of litter size (McKeowan *et al.*, 1976; Croskerry *et al.*, 1978), it is important to stress that although the body's weight is higher in the offspring of mothers treated with vitamin A, litter size remains normal. The weight increase is even more prominent in the lungs since for all the days studied, lungs from vitamin A treated fetuses are 40% heavier than the lungs of untreated fetuses, with the exception of the 17th gestational day, when the difference reaches almost 50% (Figure 6). As a result, fetal mice subjected to vitamin A supplementation present a relative lung's weight of 4,11% at the last gestational day (Figure 6). Inversely, studies performed in rats show that in the offspring of mothers with retinolemia, fetal and neonatal body weight, as well as the lung, heart and liver relative weights suffer a significant decrease when compared to control animals (Antipatis *et al.*, 1998, 2000). Maternal mild or moderate vitamin A deficiency (MVAD) in rats, where no visible clinical manifestations are registered, both in mothers and offspring, also decreases body weight and lung weight of the newborn (Wei *et al.*, 2009).

The observations carried out under light and transmission electron microscopy reveal that mice fetuses from vitamin A-treated mothers show higher lung volume and prospective branching of the respiratory tree than fetuses from untreated pregnant females. This trophic effect of vitamin A is not followed by significant changes in the normal sequence and timing of the different periods of pulmonary morphogenesis. The composition, structure, and blood vessels (in terms of the number and localization of capillary vessels) are also normal. During the intermediate periods of lung development (canalicular and early saccular stages), lungs subjected to the influence of vitamin A are denser and less saccular than lungs developing under physiological conditions. This is caused by an increase in the number of tubular and saccular structures, corresponding to heavier lungs registered in vitamin A treated fetuses. The effect of vitamin A maternal administration is particularly evident upon fetuses on the last gestational day and at the day of birth (Figure 7), where a much higher branching degree of the tubular structures is seen. This terminal tubules and saccules display an epithelium composed of type II penumocytes, which show active synthesis and excretion of multilamellar bodies (Figure 8) and flat cells in obvious scamous differentiation unto type I pneumocytes. Moreover, in the lung's instersticium, that will give rise to the primary septa, there seems to be a higher number of cells displaying lipid droplets, suggesting an increase of lipid interstitial cells or lipofibroblasts (Figure 9). This is not surpising taking into account that in adults the number of lipofibroblasts can be increased by the administration of retinyl palmitate (Chytil, 1992; McGowan *et al.,* 1995), and that these cells store retinyl (Spit, 1983; Okabe *et al.*, 1984). Furthermore, lipofibroblasts express tropoelastin (the core protein of the elastic fibers) in response to endogenous or exogenous exposure to retinoids (McGowan *et al.*, 1997), a fact that suggests an enhancement of elastogenesis in the lungs of vitamin A treated fetuses. Lipofibroblasts also store triglycerides, which are used for surfactant phospholipd synthesis in the neighboring type II pneumocytes (Torday *et al.*, 1995).

Taken together, the biometric and morphological data herein reported, lead to the conclusion that fetuses developed under the influence of vitamin A display a well developed respiratory tree, particularly in the most distal portions, with a lining of surfactant-producing cells, flat cells, intersacular septa with a good capillary network, and the presence of lipid- and vitamin A-storing interstitial cells (lipid intersticial cells), which are all aspects that favor the maturation of the lung and an enhanced alveolarization, which in mice as in humans takes place predominantly after birth.

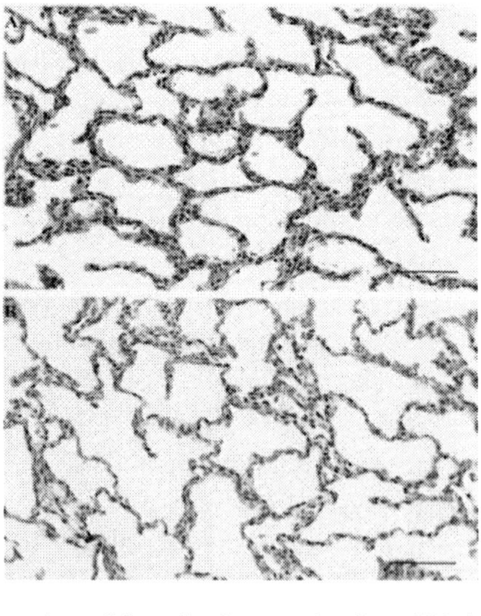

Figure 7. Histological section of the mice lung at the day of birth (approximately 4 hours of life). Notice the presence of alveolar sacs and true alveoli with well-developed septa in the lungs of vitamin-A-treated newborns (A). In control animals (B) the alveolar sacs are primitive, are limited by thin underdeveloped septa, and there is an absence of true alveoli. H-E; Scale bars=100μm.

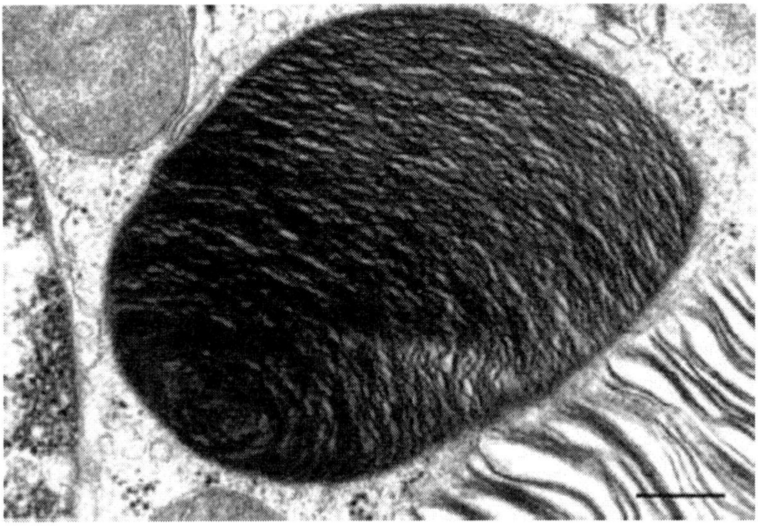

Figure 8. Transmission electron micrograph of a multilamellar body in the cytoplasm of an alveolar epithelial type II cell (pneumocyte type II). Scale bar=0.5μm.

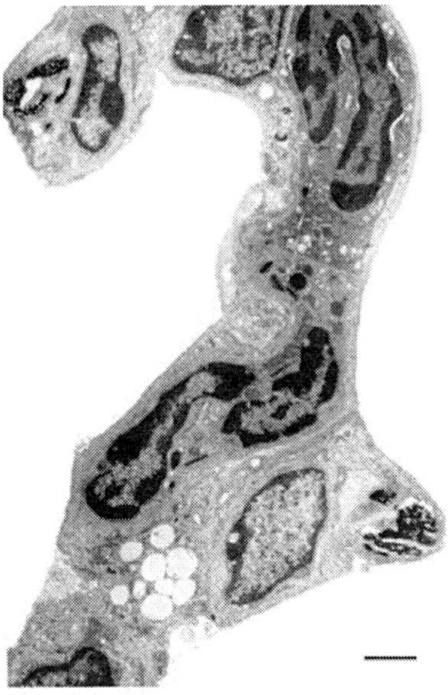

Figure 9. Transmission electron micrograph of a lipofibroblast in the alveolar septa. Scale bar=2μm.

Chapter VI

Vitamin A and Lung's Elastic Fibers

As stated before, elastic fibers have long been known to play a pivotal role in normal septal development throughout the process of lung alveolization (Burri, 1991). In order to better understand the effects of vitamin A during lung morphogenesis, our group made a morphometric and biochemical study of the lung's elastic fibers after a single subcutaneous administration of vitamin A to pregnant mice at the 14th day of gestation. In this study, the percentage of area occupied by the elastic fibers in histological sections, as well as the fraction of area filled by the alveolar septa were quantified in the newborn and at the 3rd, 5th, 8th, 10th, 14th, 15th, 17th, 21st, and 30th post-natal days. At birth, the fraction of area occupied by the elastic fibers in the lungs of animals developed under normal physiological conditions corresponds to 8% of the total area of the fields observed (Figure 10A). From this day onwards, the fraction of area occupied by the elastic fibers increases gradually and it reaches a maximum of 16.5% by the 17th post-natal day, then stabilizing to 13% in the lungs of young adults (30 days of life), by the end of the alveolarization period. On the other hand, in the lungs of animals subjected to the influence of vitamin A, the values obtained for the fraction of area occupied by the elastic fibers double the values registered in the lungs of untreated animals (Figure 10B). Until 16th post-natal day, the fraction of area occupied by the elastic fibers is consistently and statistically significant higher in vitamin A treated animals. Howeveron the 21st post-natal day the values were similar for both groups and represented 13% of the total area of the fields observed. The estimation of elastin concentration in the lungs was obtained through the chemical determination of desmosines and isodesmosines by high pressure liquid chromatography (HPLC) analysis, and revealed a positive strong correlation with the values registered in the morphometric study. Until the 15th post-natal day, the values of total elastin in the lungs developed under the influence of vitamin A are higher than the ones observed in untreated animals (Figure 11). These findings are probably related to the higher activity of lipofibroblasts, induced by the administration of vitamin A, since mice that have a null delection of RARγ, and lack one allele of RXRα, have diminished transcripts for tropoelastin in their lipofibroblasts at the post-natal day 10 and contain less elastin in their lungs at post-natal day 28, indicating that RA mediates up-regulation of elastin (McGowan *et al.*, 2000).

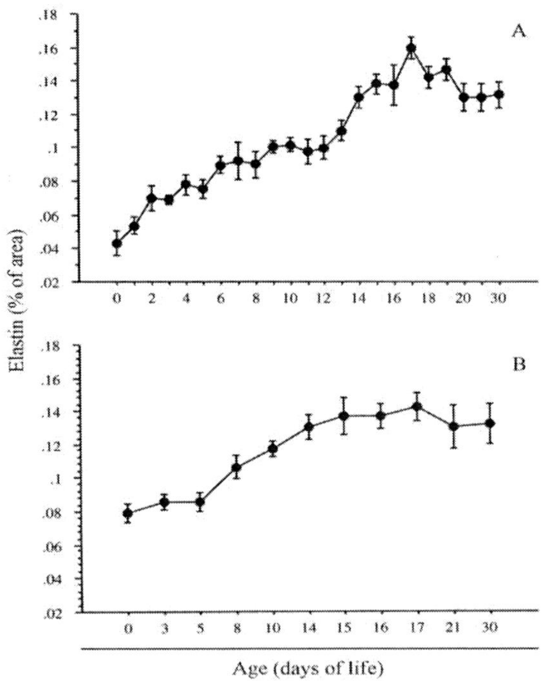

Figure 10. Fraction of area occupied by the elastic fibers in the mice lung during the first 30 days of life expressed in percentage (mean ± SD). The fraction of area occupied by the elastic fibers in the lungs of animals developed under normal physiological conditions (A) increases gradually until the 17th postnatal day, after which it stabilizes reaching 13% of the total area of the fields observed. Until the 16th day, the fraction of area occupied by the elastic fibers is consistently higher in animals exposed to vitamin A during gestation (B), but decreases afterwards, and at the 21st day of life the percentages of area are similar in both groups.

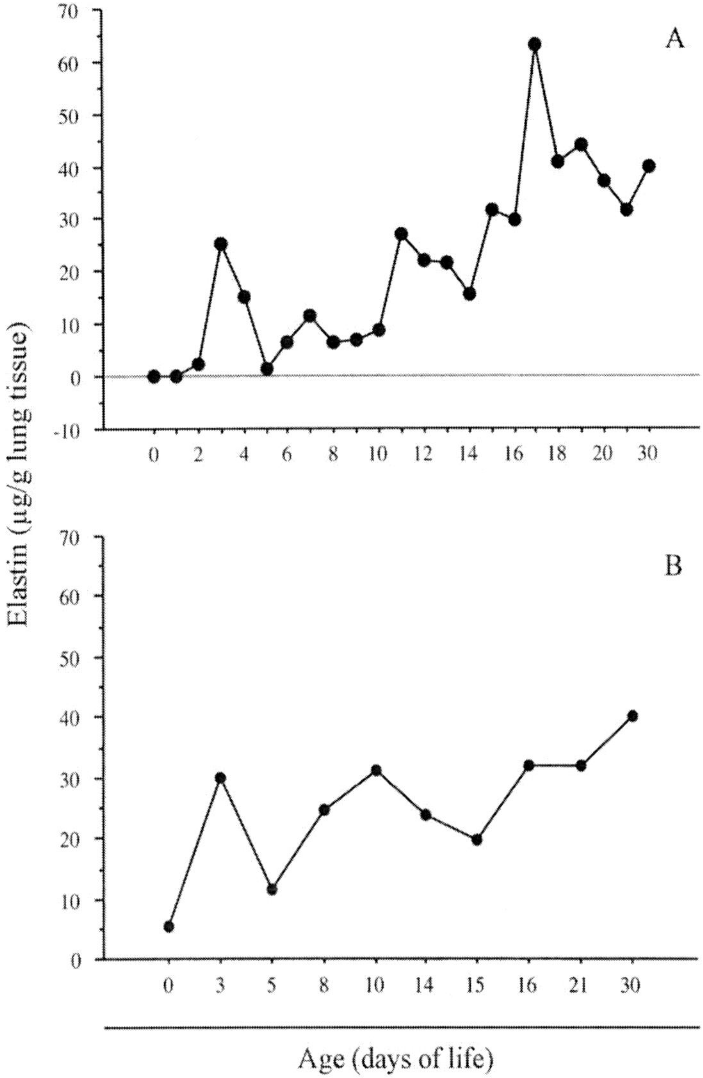

Figure 11. Elastin concentration in the mice lung during the first 30 days of life expressed in µg/g of lung tissue (mean ± SD). Animals not subjected to vitamin A influence (A) have much lower elastin values when compared to vitamin-A-treated animals (B), especially during the first 15 days of life.

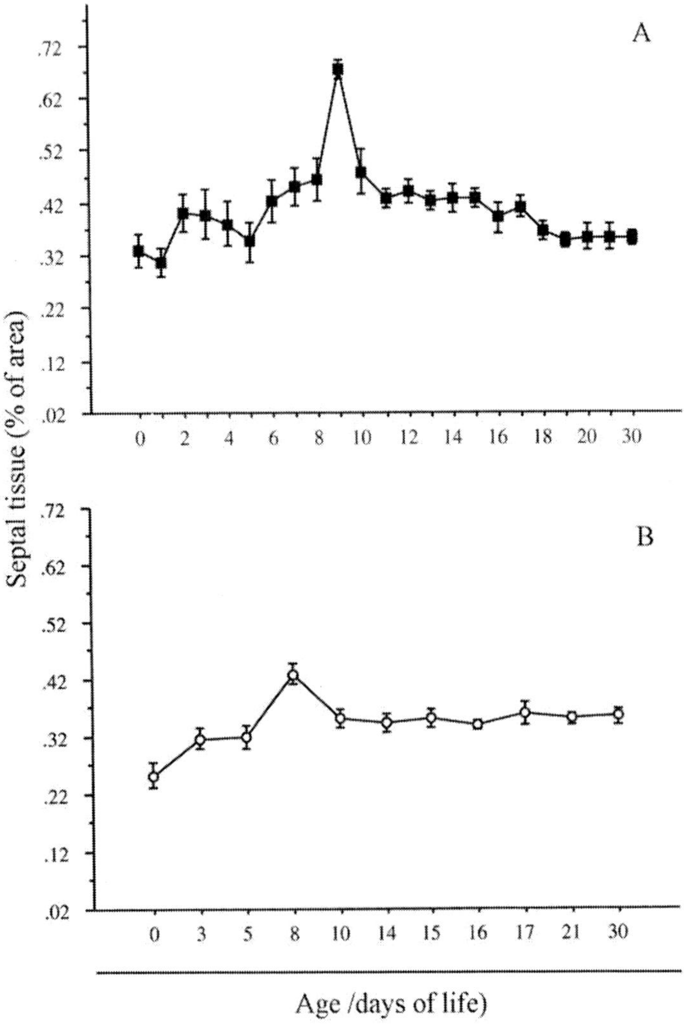

Figure 12. Fraction of area occupied by the septal tissue (alveolar septa) in the mice lung during the first 30 days of life expressed in percentage (mean ± SD). In animals developed under physiological conditions, the thickness of the alveolar septa stabilizes at the postnatal day 18, while in animals exposed to vitamin A during gestation the stabilization of the septal tissue occurs earlier, at postnatal day 10 (B).

The fraction of the area occupied by the primary and secondary septa, where the elastic fibers were analyzed and quantified, was also assessed during the time period mentioned before. At birth, the fraction of the area occupied by the septa constitutes 27% of the total area of the observed fields (Figure 12).

From this day onwards the values observed are variable, although there is an overall tendency to an in increase up till the post-natal day 8, at which time point the area occupied by the septa covers 42.5% of the total area. On the opposite, a gradual and sustained increase of the fraction of the area occupied by the septa occurs in the lungs of vitamin A treated animals that at birth corresponds to 32.5% of the total area, and is higher than the one observed in the lungs of untreated animals. Interestingly, the offspring of rats with MVAD during gestation has fewer alveoli, reduced total alveolar surface area, and increased alveolar septa thickness with increased collagen deposits and decreased elastic fibers. However, early post-natal vitamin A supplementation can restore the normal lung structure (Wei *et al.*, 2009). Together with these findings, the morphological study also performed by our group leads clearly to the conclusion that the administration of vitamin A speeds up the process of pulmonary alveolization, which is accompanied by an anticipation of the appearance of the elastic fibers at the level of the lung's respiratory portion. Again, mice that have a null delection of RARγ, and lack one allele of RXRα display a reduction in alveolar and the gas/exchange surface area (McGowan *et al.*, 2000), thus illustrating the pivotal role of RA in the alveolization process.

Chapter VII

Vitamin A and Its Derivatives during Gestation and in the Postnatal Period

During gestation, maternal vitamin A status has a profound impact on fetal growth and development. When circulating levels of retinoids are reduced in pregnant rats, a disruption between the real gestational time and the corresponding fetal development occurs (Antipatis *et al.*, 1998, 2000). Additionally, plasma retinol concentrations are lower (Hustead *et al.*, 1984; Verma *et al.*, 1996; Inder *et al.*, 1998) and hepatic stores less (Shenai *et al.*, 1990; Zachman *et al.*, 1996) in pre-term infants that develop bronchopulmonary dysplasia, supporting the hypothesis that vitamin A deficiency contributes to the development of chronic lung disease and/or respiratory tract infections in this population. Moreover, in rats, the plasma retinol concentrations of both mother and offspring are reduced by approximately 40% in MVAD (Wei *et al.*, 2009).

The effect of a charge of vitamin A on the distribution of retinol and retinyl palmitate in the mother's plasma, liver, lung, placenta, amniotic fluid, and milk, as well as in the liver and lung of fetuses was investigated by chemical quantification through HPLC. By resorting to the same analytical approach the retinol and retinyl palmitate values of the newborn mice's gastric fluid along the beast-feeding period (post-natal day 17), which made possible to know the concentration of vitamin A in the mother's milk, were determined. The retinol and retinyl palmitate levels of the liver from birth up to the 30th day of life were also assessed. For the fetal studies, pregnant mice received a single subcutaneous injection of vitamin A on the 12th day of gestation, while for the postnatal studies vitamin A was administered at the 14th gestational day.

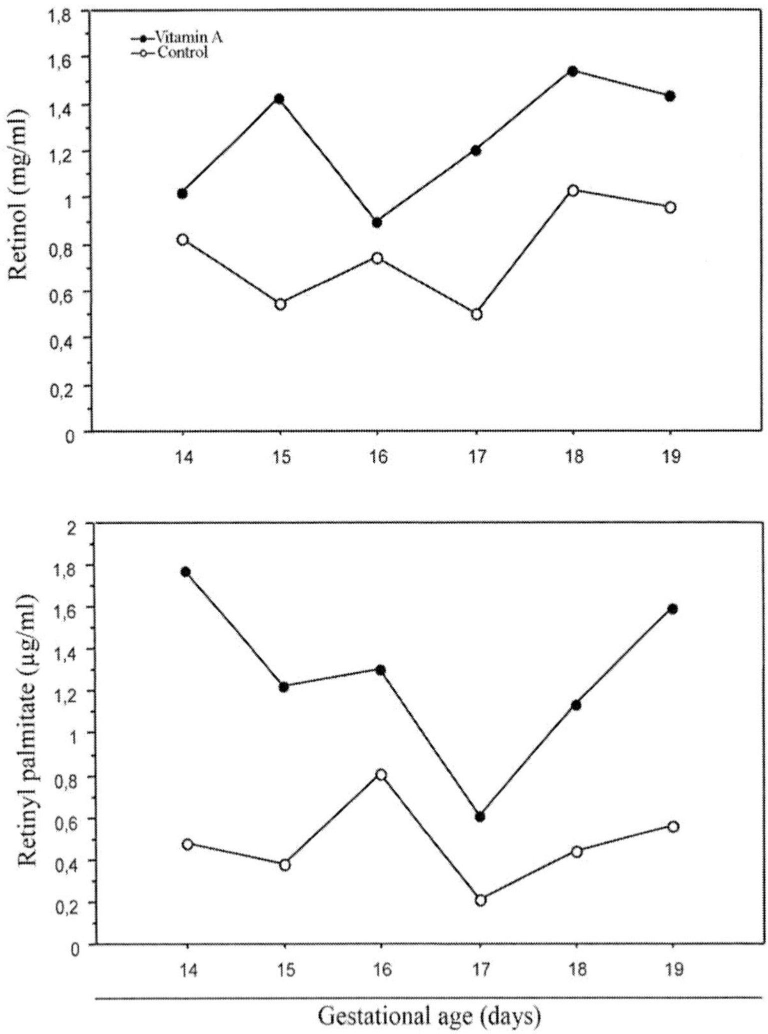

Figure 13. Retinol and retinyl palmitate plasmatic concentration in female pregnant mice expressed in µg/ml (mean ± SD). During normal gestation both retinoids suffer only slight variations but are increased in females injected with vitamin A.

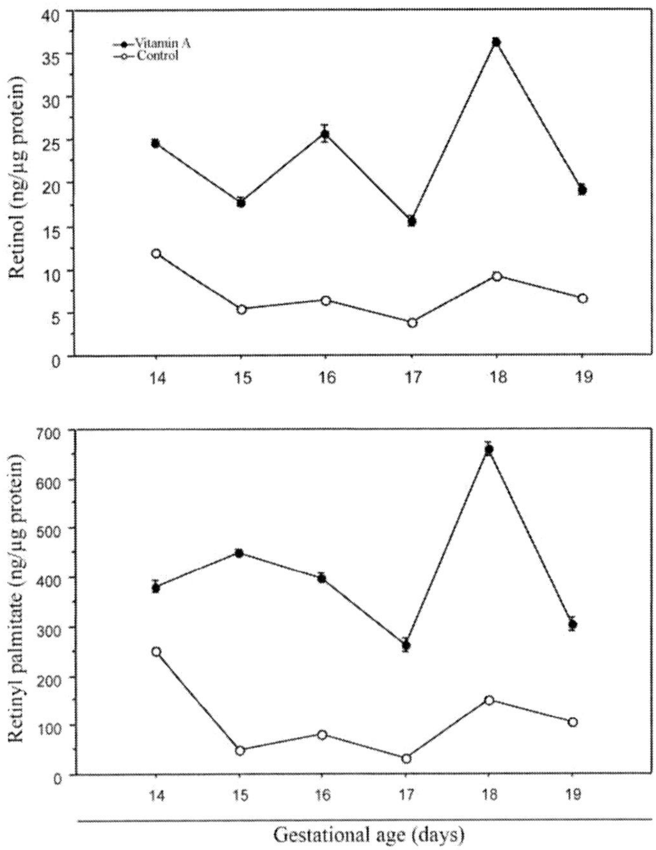

Figure 14. Retinol and retinyl palmitate concentration in the liver of female pregnant mice expressed in µg/µg of protein (mean ± SD). Retinol and retinyl palmitate hepatic levels are highest at the 14th gestational day in females not supplemented with vitamin A, while females exposed to this micronutrient display higher values of both retinoids through out the gestational period. Regarding retinyl palmitate, the most prominent difference (a 837% increase) between control and injected animals take place at the 15th gestational day.

Throughout normal gestation, both plasma retinol and retinyl palmitate levels remain fairly constant (Figure 13). However, females exposed to vitamin A present a higher variation and higher retinol and retinyl palmitate values than control females. This is particularly true for the plasmatic retinyl palmitate concentration, which displays an approximately 3-fold increase during the gestational period. Some 90% of the body's reserve of vitamin A is stored in the liver as retinyl esters, but the lung is one of the other sites of major vitamin A storage (Mactier & Weaver, 2005). As such, determining the storage capacity of these organs during normal and vitamin A-supplemented gestation is crucial. Retinol hepatic concentration peaks at the 14th gestational day (12.11 ng of retinol per each μg of total protein) and reaches the lowest value at the 17th gestational day (Figure 14).

Retinol concentration is increased by 105% in the liver of mothers that received vitamin A at the 14th gestational day, and by 310% at the 17th gestational day. Retinyl palmitate hepatic values are high and display the same type of variation observed in the retinol values during gestation (Figure 14). At the 14th gestational day, retinyl palmitate levels suffer a 52% increase in the liver of mothers treated with vitamin A, and a striking 837% increase at the 15th gestational day. Retinol concentration in the lungs of pregnant mice peaks at the 17th gestational day (Figure 15). Retinyl palmitate levels in the lungs of pregnant mice range from 49.18 ng of retinyl palmitate per each μg of total protein at the 15th gestational day to 200.6 g of retinyl palmitate per each μg of total protein at the following day (Figure 15).

Retinyl palmitate values are significantly higher and correlate negatively with those of retinol in the lungs of pregnant mice injected with vitamin A, both retinol and retinyl palmitate concentrations suffer a significant increase through out the entire gestational period, when compared to control pregnant females. This effect is even more pronounced in the retinyl palmitate content. Regarding the placenta, retinol values in mothers not exposed to vitamin A range from 0.361 ng of retinol per each μg of total protein at the 14th gestational day to 0.582 ng of retinol per each μg of total protein at the 17th day of gestation (Figure 16).

Females injected with vitamin A however, show a significant increase of the placental retinol levels, when compared to control animals. On the other hand, retinyl palmitate concentration in the placenta of control animals is barely detectable at the 14th day of gestation (0.05 ng of retinyl palmitate per each μg of total protein) and peaks at the 15th gestational day (0.123 of retinyl palmitate per each μg of total protein).

Similarly to the observed for the placental retinol content, retinyl palmitate values in the placenta of females that received vitamin A are clearly superior to those obtained in control mothers. In the amniotic fluid, retinol concentration is low and remains relatively constant until the end of gestation (Figure 17), but increases 2.5- to 15-fold by vitamin A administration. Retinyl palmitate levels in normal gestations range from 10.99 ng of retinyl palmitate per each μg of total protein at the 17th gestational day to 20,61 ng of retinyl palmitate per each μg of total protein at the last gestational day (Figure 17). As it happens with the retinol concentration during gestation, retinyl palmitate in the amniotic fluid is also increased by vitamin A administration. In the fetal mice lung, retinol and retinyl palmitate increase concurrently from the 14th to the 16th day of gestation, after which they slightly decrease, and then peak at the last gestational day (Figure 18). Vitamin A administration increases both retinol and retinyl palmitate levels into an extent that retinyl palmitate levels show a 3-fold (16, 18, and 19 gestational days) and a 6-fold (14, 15, and 17 gestational days) increase in the mice fetal lung.

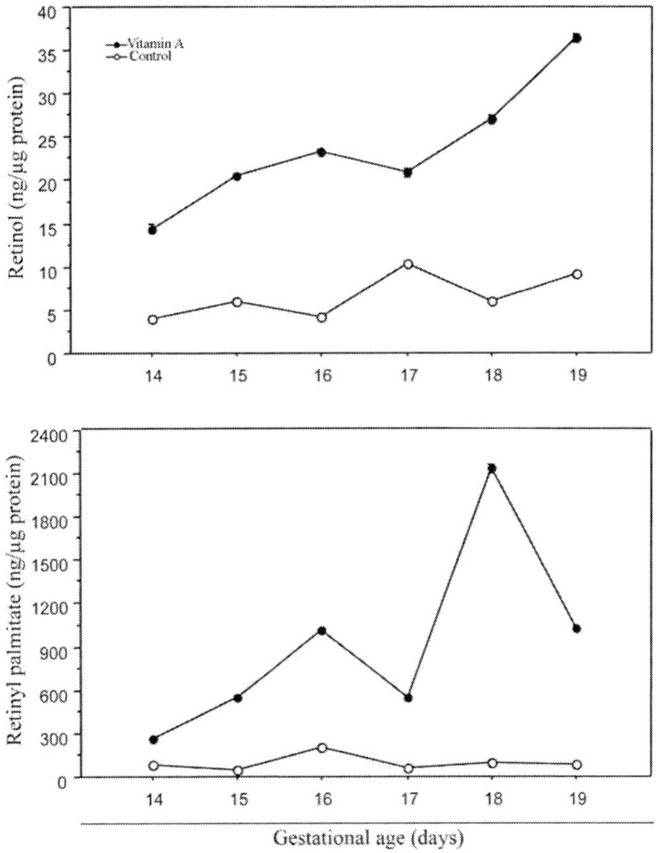

Figure 15. Retinol and retinyl palmitate concentration in the lung of female pregnant mice expressed in μg/μg of protein (mean ± SD). During normal gestation retinol and retinyl palmitate concentration in the lungs remain fairly constant, reaching a maximum at the 17th and 16th gestational days, respectively. However, in vitamin A treated females lung's retinoid storage capacity is enhanced and retinol and retinyl palmitate concentration are highest at the end of gestation.

In fetuses developed under physiological conditions, both retinol and retinyl palmitate liver content increases gradually from the 14th until the 16th gestational days, then decreases slightly at day 17, but increases again until the end of gestation (Figure 19). Albeit markedly higher than those registered in control fetuses, retinol and retinyl palmitate values in the liver of fetuses from vitamin A treated mothers display the same overall tendency during the gestational period. This aspect is not present during the postnatal period.

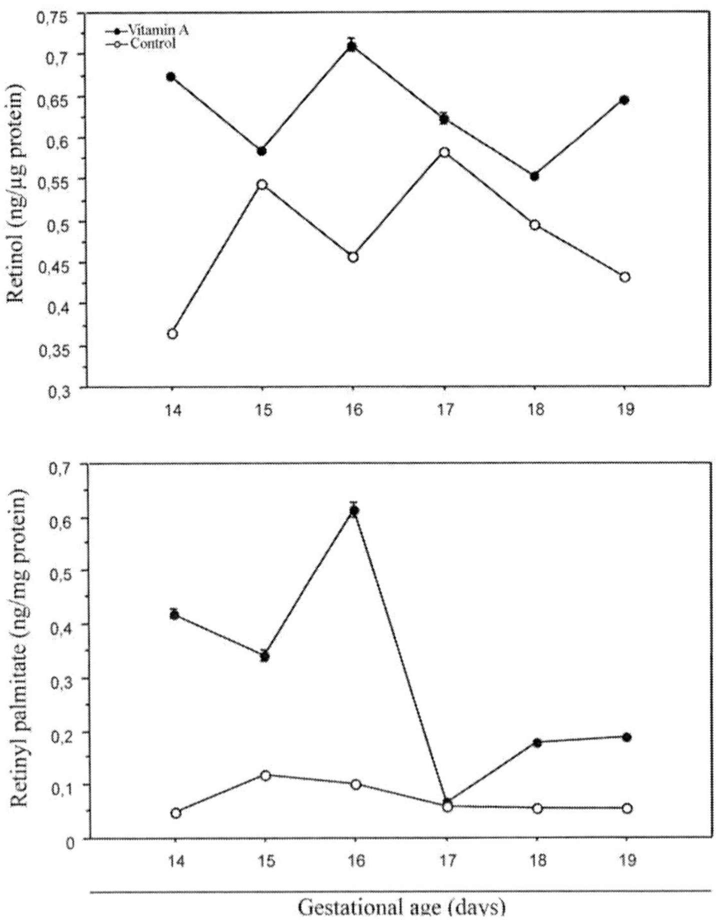

Figure 16. Retinol and retinyl palmitate concentration in the placenta of female pregnant mice expressed in ng/µg of protein for retinol and ng/mg of protein for retinyl palmitate (mean ± SD). Females exposed to vitamin A present higher values of retinol and retinyl palmitate in the placenta that peak at the 16th gestational day. During normal gestation retinyl palmitate values in the placenta are extremely low.

During the first 30 days of life, both retinol and retinyl palmitate hepatic concentration varies greatly (Figures 20 A and 21 A), but the values are persistently lower than the ones observed in the adult (8 and 1200 μg per each gram of liver tissue, respectively). At birth, retinol liver values in the animals subjected to vitamin A during gestation triple the values registered in control animals. By the 5th day of life, retinol hepatic levels in vitamin A treated animals reach a maximum of 5 μg per each gram of liver tissue, but decline gradually into a point that they are similar to those of control animals by the end of the first month of age (Figure 20 B). Newborn exposed to vitamin A during gestation present a 13-fold increase in the retinyl palmitate liver content, which peaks at the postnatal day 5, and then declines to values close to the ones observed in the liver of control animals at postnatal day 30 (Figure 21 B). During the fetal period it is important to notice that the retinoid content in the lung and liver declines abruptly at the 17th gestational day, which indicates the occurrence of profound modifications in the retinoid metabolism and homeostasis, and suggests the possible mobilization of lung and hepatic retinoid storages crucial for fetal development and organogenesis.

During the first 15 days of life, mice's gastric fluid is exclusively composed of maternal milk and contains reduced quantities of retinol (Figure 22 A), which suffer discrete increases by the 4th, 8th, and 14th postnatal days. Likewise, retinyl palmitate levels in the mice's gastric fluid are very low and proved impossible to quantify through the methods used in the first 48 hours of life (Figure 23 A). Approximately 4 hours after birth, the retinol content in the gastric fluid of animals exposed to vitamin A is 10 times higher than in control animals (Figure 22 B), after which it falls abruptly at postnatal day 3, then increases slightly at day 5 and remains relatively constant until the 17th day of life. In the same animals, retinyl palmitate levels in the mice's gastric fluid are high (19.5 g of retinyl palmitate per for each gram of gastric fluid), but also decline at postnatal day 3. Even so, they remain 3 times higher than the ones registered in control animals (Figure 23 B).

Throughout pregnancy, maternal mechaninsms of vitamin A homeostasis are mobilized to ensure that adequate levels of retinoids are available and reach the embryo and fetus through accurate mechanisms of transplacental transfer. Nevertheless, given the fundamental role of retinoids in embryonic development it is of vital importance that the conceptus should form its autonomous vitamin A reserves and can be capable of maintaining normal levels of this compound. Sadly, vitamin A sufficiency cannot be assumed for pre-term infants. This significant subgroup of our infant population is born with inadequate body stores of vitamin A, is often unable to tolerate routine oral supplementation, and is prone to diseases of the eye and respiratory and gastrointestinal tracts. Compared to term infants, preterm infants have low plasma concentrations of both retinol and retinol binding protein (RBP) at birth, which remain low during the infant's stay in the neonatal unit, and throughout the first year of life (Mactier & Weaver, 2005).

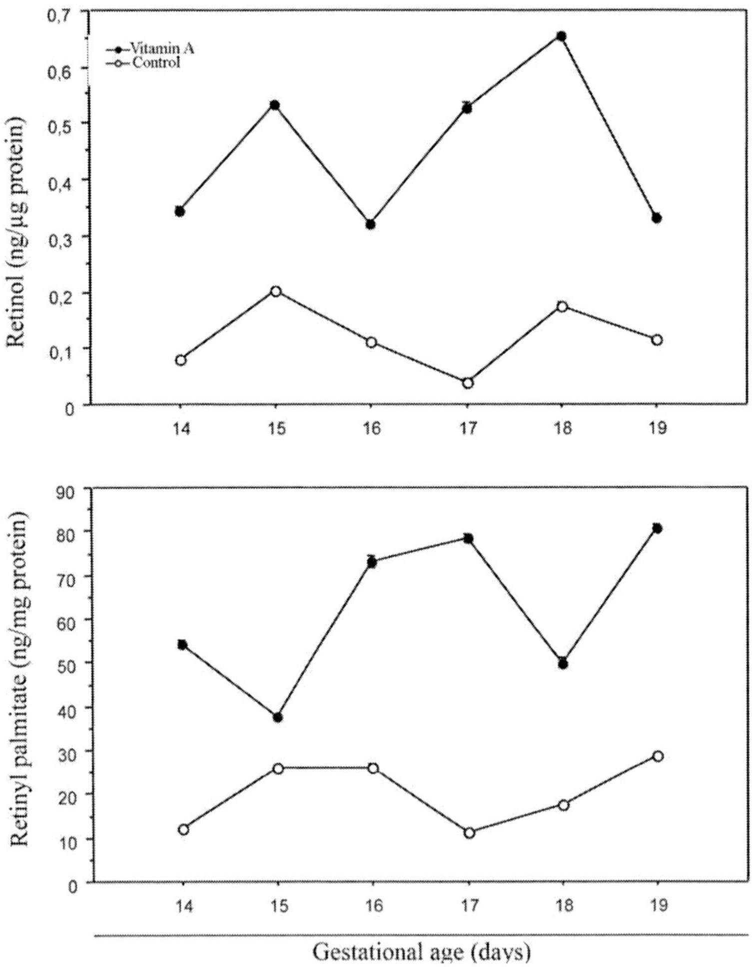

Figure 17. Retinol and retinyl palmitate concentration in the amniotic fluid of mice expressed in ng/μg of protein for retinol and ng/mg of protein for retinyl palmitate (mean ± SD). In normal gestations, retinol levels are low in the amniotic fluid and remain constant through out the gestational period, however vitamin A administration increases their concentration. Retinyl palmitate concentration in the amniotic fluid peaks at the last gestational day and is also enhanced by vitamin A exposure.

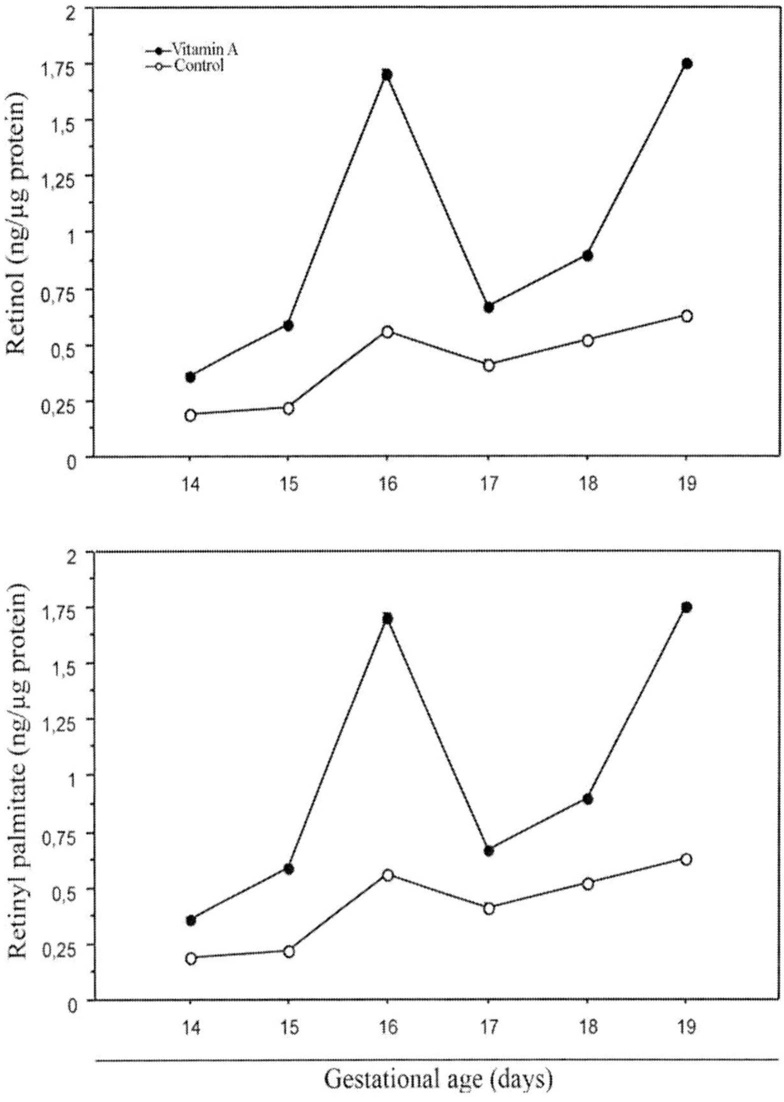

Figure 18. Retinol and retinyl palmitate concentration in the lungs of fetal mice expressed in μg/μg of protein (mean ± SD). Both retinoids increase concurrently from the 14th to the 16th day of gestation, after which they slightly decrease, and then peak at the last gestational day. Fetuses exposed Vitamin A show higher values of retinol and retinyl palmitate in their lungs.

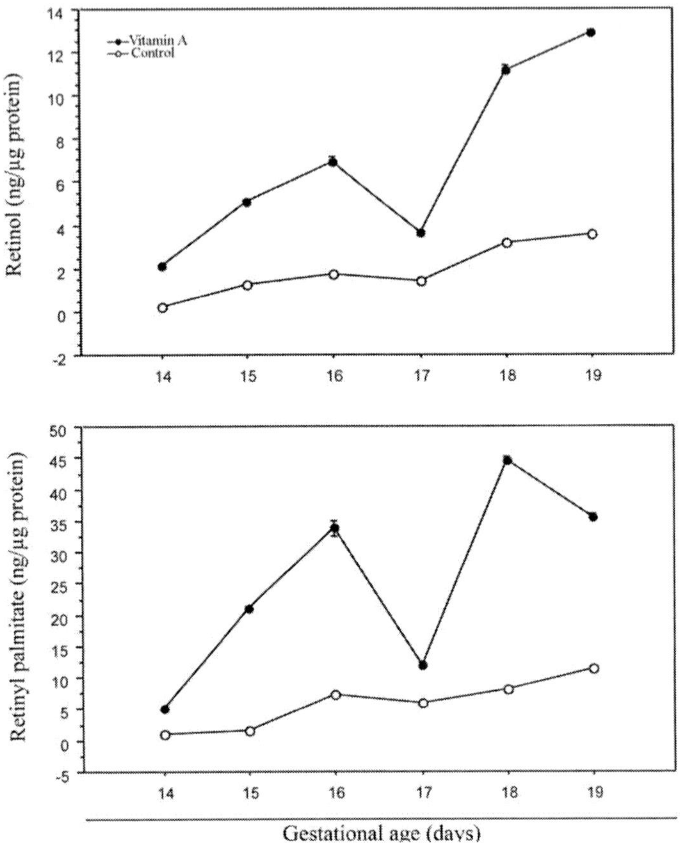

Figure 19. Retinol and retinyl palmitate concentration in the liver of fetal mice expressed in μg/μg of protein (mean ± SD). Both retinoids increase gradually from the 14th until the 16th gestational days, then decrease slightly at day 17, but increase again until the end of gestation. Vitamin A administration doesn't alter this overall tendency but increases the liver's retinoid storage capacity.

Our studies provided evidence that from the 14th gestational day till birth, all analyzed tissues, including maternal plasma and amniotic fluid, show responsiveness to the administration of vitamin A. At the same time, fetal tissues, as well as the amniotic fluid, display from an early age an important storage capacity for retinyl palmitate. These reserves may be useful in the case of the fall of the mother's retilonemia or deficiency in the transplacental transfer of retinoids. The hepatic storage capacity of retinoids is also enhanced in animals exposed to vitamin A during the postnatal period. Furthermore, the biochemical analysis of the newborn mice's gastric fluid leads to the conclusion that the mothers injected with vitamin A during pregnancy excrete through the milk and mostly during the days immediately after birth quantities of retinol and retinyl palmitate that are largely superior (1.6 mg of retinol and 20 mg of retinyl palmitate for each gram of gastric fluid at birth) to those excreted in the milk of female pregnant mice not submitted to vitamin A administration (0.1 mg of retinol and undetectable values of retinyl palmitate for each gram of gastric fluid at birth), thus acting as a natural supplementation of this nutrient.

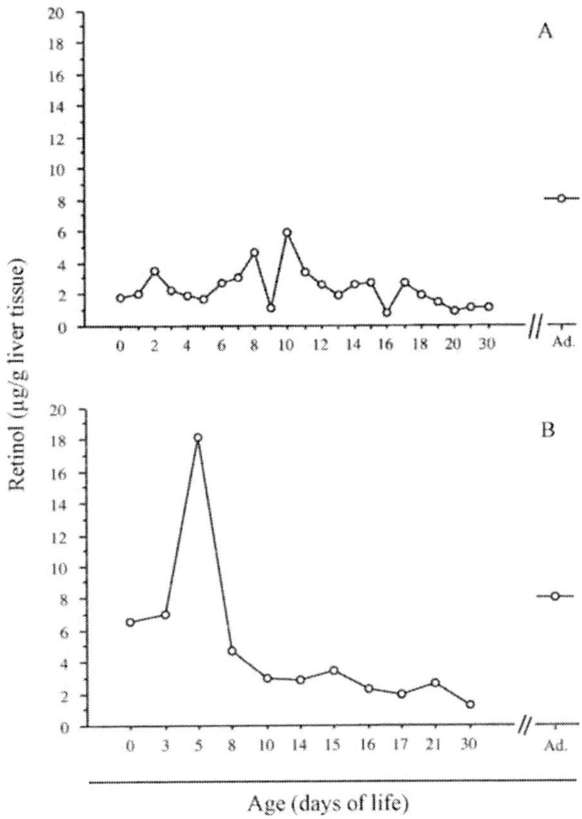

Figure 20. Retinol concentration in the liver of mice during the first 30 days of life expressed in µg/µg of liver tissue (mean ± SD). In animals developed under physiological conditions (A) retinol hepatic values suffer variations, especially during the first 16 days of life. Administration of vitamin A during gestation (B) results in an increase of retinol hepatic concentration in the postnatal period, reaching a maximum at the 5th postnatal day, after which time point it declines gradually and becomes similar to those of control animals by the end of the first month of age. Ad.: normal value in the adult.

Chapter VIII

Vitamin A and Its Derivatives in the Adult

Two decades ago, an association between serum vitamin A levels and lung function in patients with chronic obstructive lung disease (COPD) suggested an involvement of RA signaling in lung homeostasis (Morabia *et al.*, 1990), but since then it has long been established that the adult lung responds to RA administration.

The first report to attest this fact was performed by Massaro and Massaro (1997), who clearly demonstrated that RA is able to fully or partially rescue emphysema-like lesions induced by the intratracheal instillation of elastase. A similar effect of RA is also seen in the tight-skin mutant mouse, which has a genetic failure of alveolar development, and in post-natal rats treated with dexamethsone (Massaro *et al.*, 2000). More recently, other studies showed that when administered to adult mice, RA restores the lung cytoarchitecture that had previously been disrupted by the postnatal administration of dexamethasone (Hind & Maden, 2004). However, not all the retinoids have the same efficacy on alveolar regeneration in the dexamethasone treated models. For example, retinol alone is not effective in alveolar repair, while transRA and a RARα agonist successfully induce alveolar regeneration (Maden, 2006).

More curiously, not all studies have show that RA can rescue alveolar regeneration in lung injury different models. Some have shown only a partial rescue of alveolar surface area (Tepper *et al.*, 2000).Other sources have in fact failed to show benefits of RA in emphysema lesions (Srinivasan *et al.*, 2002; Lucey *et al.*, 2003; Fujita *et al.*, 2004; March *et al.*, 2004, 2005). One of the reasons that could explain these apparently contradictory results is the difference in RA pharmacokinetics between strains and species. Our work was centered on the effect of vitamin A in adult mice. The studies were carried out on a daily basis during the first 14 days after the administration of vitamin A and then on a fortnightly one up to the 90th day. The pulmonary concentration of retinol and retynil palmitate, as well as the corresponding plasmatic and hepatic levels, was analyzed through HPLC.

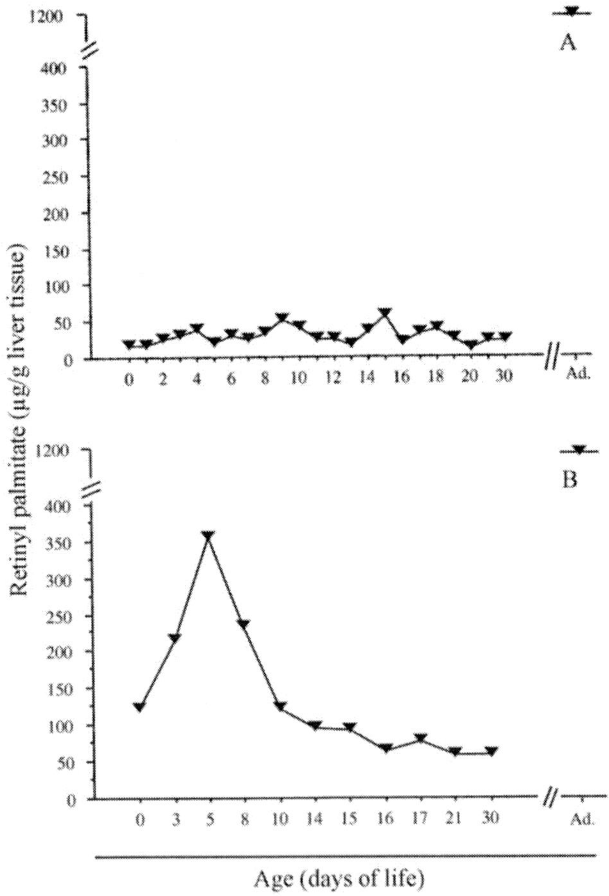

Figure 21. Retinyl palmitate concentration in the liver of mice during the first 30 days of life expressed in µg/µg of liver tissue (mean ± SD). Despite its variations during the first month of age retinyl palmitate concentration in the liver is persistently lower than in the adult (A). Vitamin A administration (B) increases retinyl palmitate hepatic levels that are at birth 13 times higher than the values registered in the liver of control animals. Ad.: normal value in the adult.

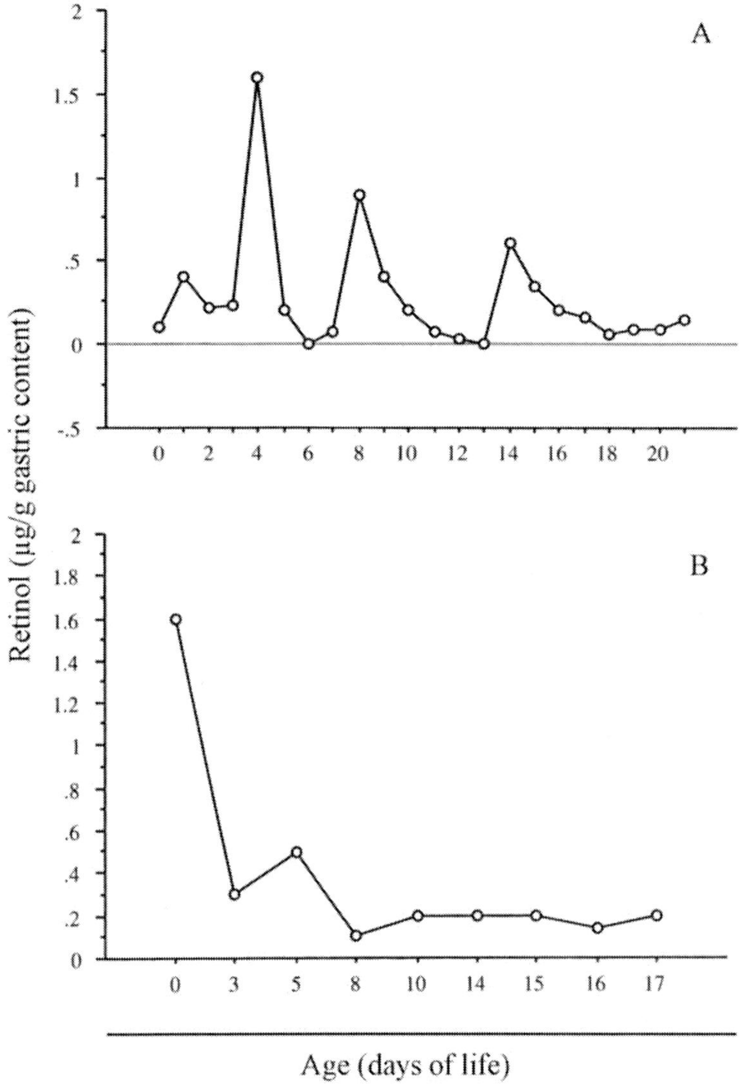

Figure 22. Retinol concentration in the gastric content of mice during the first 30 days of life expressed in µg/g of gastric content (mean ± SD). Retinol values are very low and display discrete increases by the 4th, 8th, and 14th postnatal days (A). However, exposure to vitamin A during gestation leads to an increase of retinol in the gastric fluid (B), which at birth is 10 times higher in treated animals when compare to control subjects.

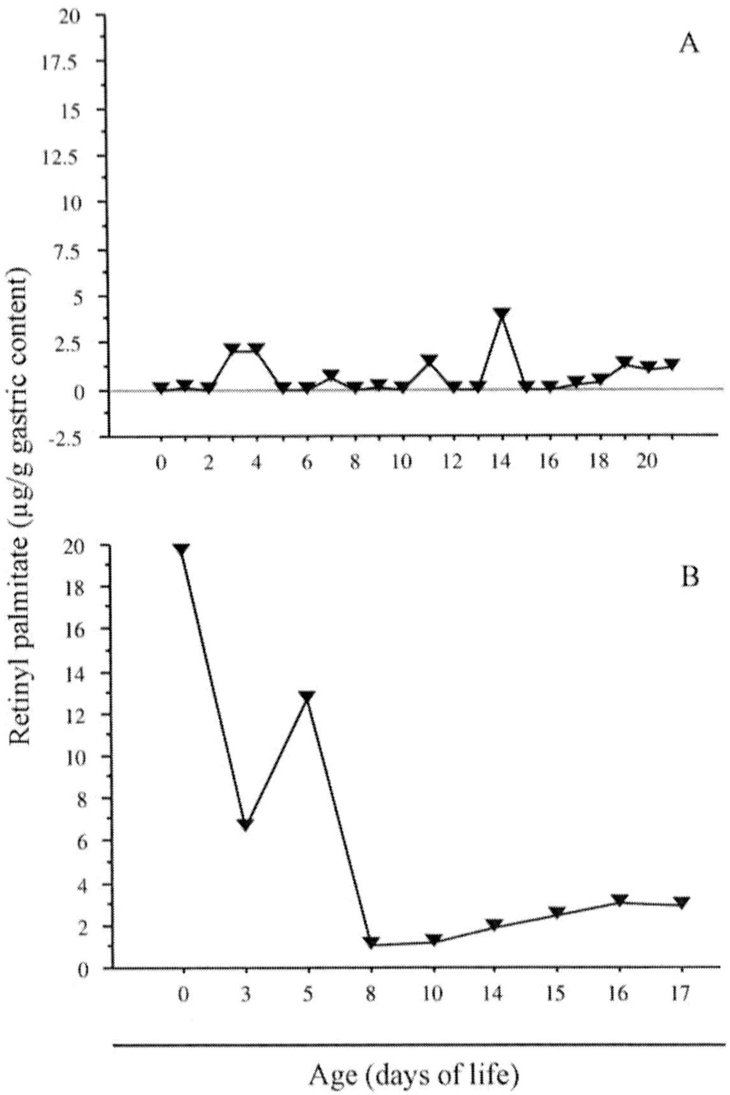

Figure 23. Retinyl palmitate concentration in the gastric content of mice during the first 30 days of life expressed in µg/g of gastric content (mean ± SD). Retinyl palmitate quantities in the mice's gastric fluid are very low and impossible to quantify in the first 48 hours of life (A). Vitamin A administration results in an increase of retinyl palmitate concentration in the mice's gastric fluid (B), which peaks at the day of birth, declines at postnatal day 3, but remains higher than the one observed in animals developed under physiological conditions.

The morphometrical study revealed that 48 hours after the administration of vitamin A the architectural pattern of the adult lung is normal and remains that way in the following days (Figure 24), but there is a sudden septal thickening around the 8th day (Figures 25 and 26). This results from an increase of the pulmonary interstiticial cells and extracecellular material, which decreases the alveolar lumen, a morphological aspect that matches the alveolar stage of lung development. These findings are accompanied by an increase of the lipid droplets in the interstitial's cells cytoplasm (Figure 27).

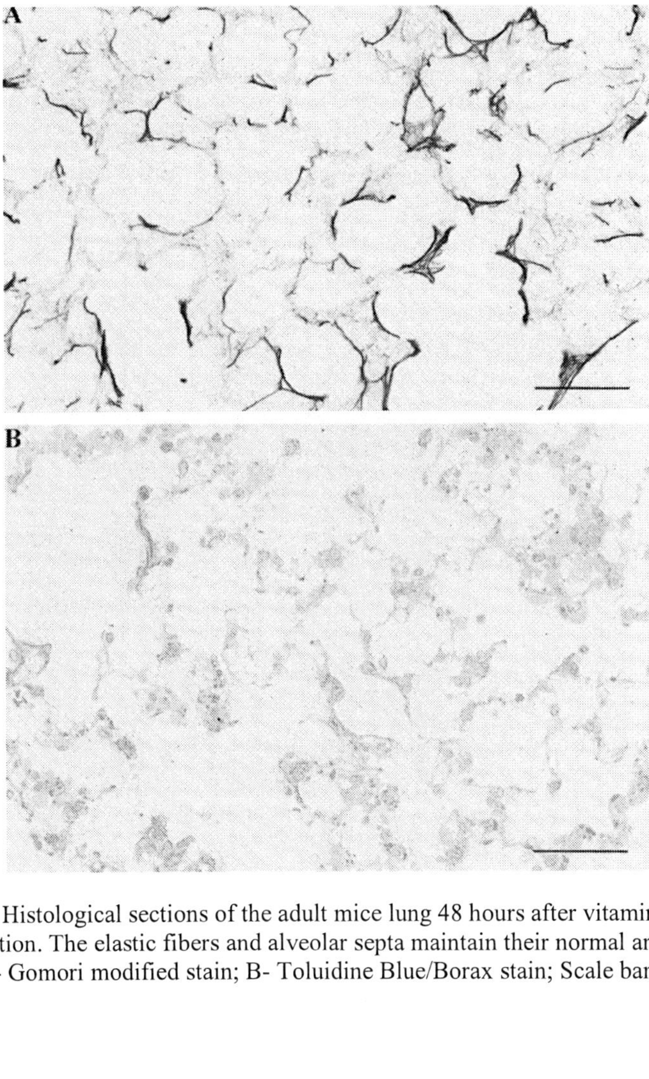

Figure 24. Histological sections of the adult mice lung 48 hours after vitamin A administration. The elastic fibers and alveolar septa maintain their normal architectural pattern. A- Gomori modified stain; B- Toluidine Blue/Borax stain; Scale bars=100μm.

From the 9th to the 12th days after vitamin A injection a gradual decrease in septal thickness is seen (Figure 25), which continues until the 90th day, when the lungs display normal morphological features. No changes are recorded with the regard to the percentage of area occupied by the elastic fibers throughout the whole period.

Retinol and retinyl palmitate plasmatic levels in the adult vary differently after a charge of vitamin A. While plasmatic retinol concentration presents minor changes during the 90 days period after vitamin A administration, retinyl palmitate plasmatic values display great differences through out the same period of time (Figure 28).

These findings are in agreement with the observations made in humans, according to which retinol plasmatic levels remain relatively constant regardless of the dietary intake of vitamin A (Blomhoff *et al.*, 1990). Despite of this, both retinol and retinyl palmitate levels are persistently higher than the ones registered in control adult animals. Vitamin A administration rapidly increases retinol levels in the lung and liver (Figure 29). In the lung, the most prominent increase takes place between the 3rd and 11th day after vitamin A injection, after which the retinol levels suffer an overall decrease, and by the 90th day of study they are similar to the basal values found in control animals.

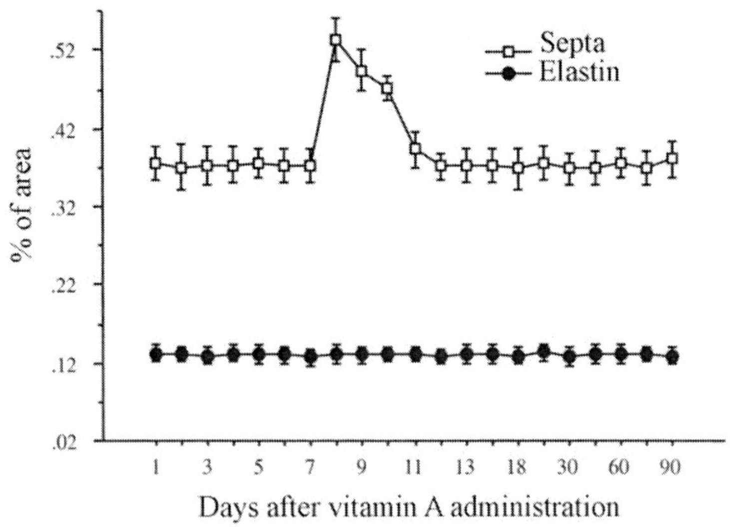

Figure 25. Fraction of area occupied by the alveolar septa and the elastic fibers during the 90 days period after vitamin A administration expressed in percentage (mean ± SD). Septal thickness is increased at postnatal days 8, 9, and 10, while no changes are seen in the fraction of area occupied by the elastic fibers.

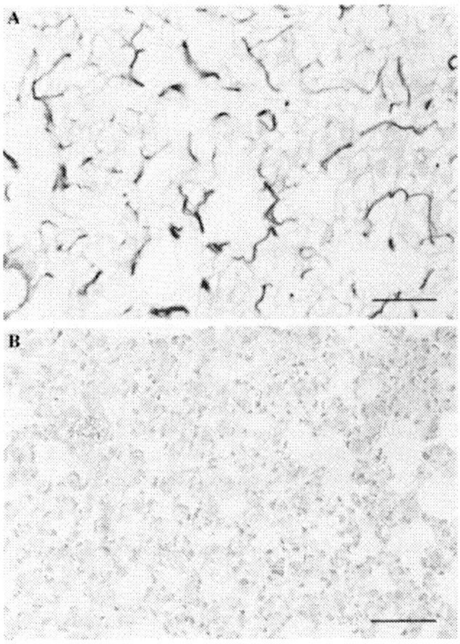

Figure 26. Histological sections of the adult mice lung 8 days after vitamin A administration. Marked septal thickening and diminished alveolar lumen that resembles the alveolar stage of lung development. A- Gomori modified stain; B- Toluidine Blue/Borax stain; Scale bars=100μm.

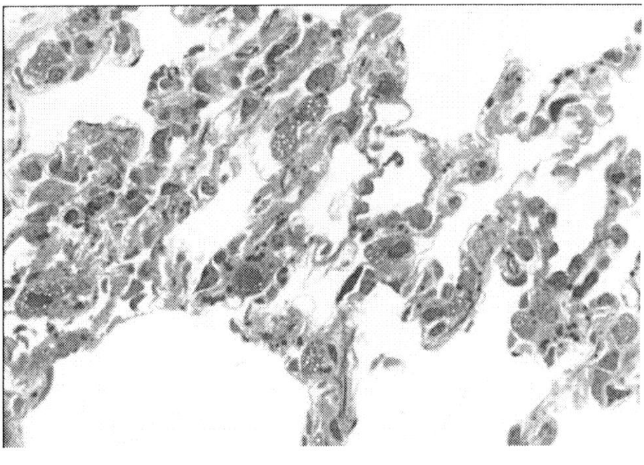

Figure 27. Histological section of the adult mice lung 8 days after vitamin A administration. Notice the alveolar septal thickness and the presence of lipid droplets in the cytoplasm of the interstitial cells (lipofibroblasts). Blue/Borax stain; Scale bar=100μm.

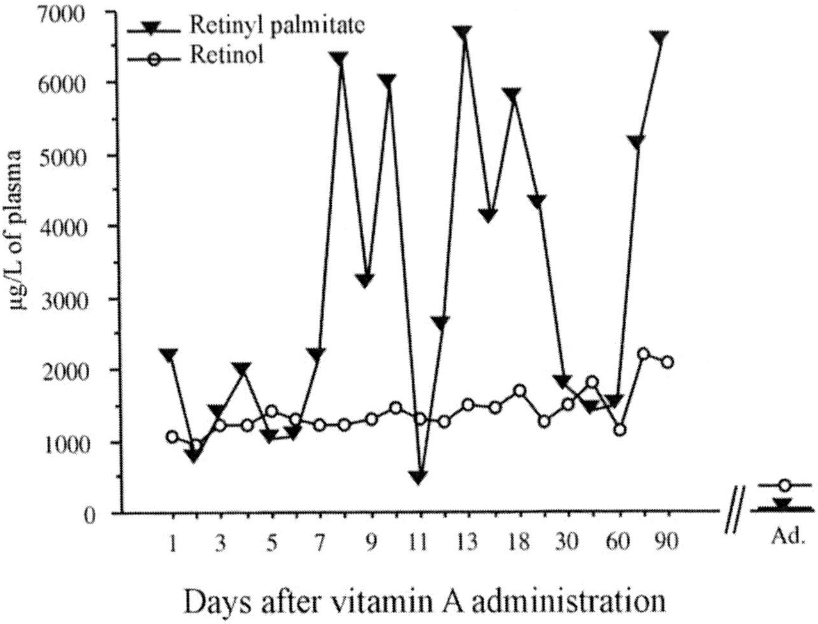

Figure 28. Retinol and retinyl palmitate plasmatic concentration in adult mice during the 90 days period after vitamin A administration expressed in µg/L. Retinol concentration presents minor changes during the period analyzed, while retinyl palmitate plasma levels vary greatly and are higher than the ones observed in the adult. Ad.: normal value in the adult.

On the other hand, retinol liver content peaks 48 hours after vitamin A injection, then declines abruptly and stabilizes until the 18th day, at which time point increases again and remains elevated until the end of study period. Regarding the retinyl palmitate levels in the lung and liver, although both organs exhibit responsiveness to vitamin A (Figure 30), it is important to stress that the lung is the first organ to react to its administration, showing a great capacity for concentrating retinyl palmitate (11 000 mg per each gram of lung tissue by the 6th day) and largely surpassing the hepatic levels (300 mg per per each gram of liver tissue by the 6th day), when considering concentration per tissue weight. This great storage and concentration capacity of vitamin A by the lung reaches its peak by the 6th day after injection and becomes unnoticeable by the 30th day.

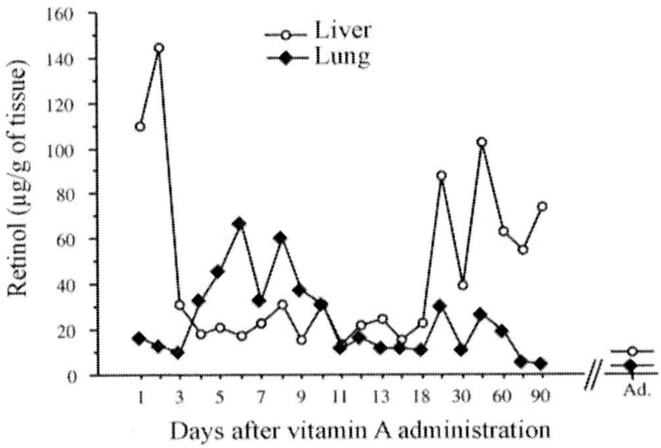

Figure 29. Retinol concentration in the liver and lungs of adult mice during the 90 days period after vitamin A administration expressed in µg/g of tissue. Vitamin A administration increases retinol hepatic and pulmonary concentration. In the lungs, a prominent increase takes place between the 3rd and 11th day after vitamin A injection, while in the liver retinol concentration reaches its maximum 48 hours after vitamin A injection, then declines abruptly and stabilizes until the 18th day, at which time point increases again and remains elevated until the end of study period. Ad.: normal value in the adult.

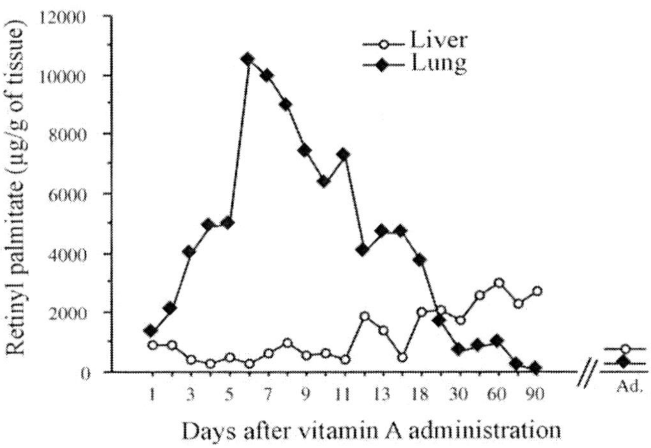

Figure 30. Retinyl palmitate concentration in the liver and lungs of adult mice during the 90 days period after vitamin A administration expressed in µg/g of tissue. Lung displays higher responsiveness to vitamin A administration, which reaches its peak 6 days after vitamin A injection. Thirty days after, retinyl palmitate concentration is similar to the normal concentration registered in the adult lung. Ad.: normal value in the adult.

Chapter IX

Lessons from Lung Injury Animal Models and Therapeutic Interventions with Vitamin A

Lung injury animal models provided useful insights on vitamin A and RA signaling pathways, some of which are mentioned in this chapter. The majority of lung injury models try, on one hand, to reproduce developmental abnormalities or, on the other hand, chronic lung diseases, such as COPD or cigarrete smoking-associated diseases. As a consequence of lung immaturity, premature newborns are at high risk of developing bronchopulmonary dysplasia (BPD); a disease characterized by vascular abnormalities and disrupted alveolarization, which compromise the whole lung maturation process. Bronchopulmonary dysplasia phatophysiology includes prolonged hyperoxia due to ventilator and oxygen therapy for acute respiratory failure after premature birth (Thébaud and Abman, 2007). This aspect motivated many investigators that concentrated efforts into the development of new therapeutic strategies and the understanding of BPD pathogenesis. Recently, a primate model of BPD revealed that postnatal vitamin A administration resulted in increased lung elastin expression, but without altering angiogenesis-related genes, namely VEGF and its receptor VEGFR2 (Pierce *et al.*, 2007). In another model of BPD, signaling between VEGF and VEGFR2 was blocked in the mice lung at postnatal day 3, which resulted in inhibited alveolarization with large, simplified alveolar structures and sparse, dysmorphic, and dilated capillaries. In this model, treatment with RA maintained alveolar surface area, mean alveolar volume, and volume density of endothelial cells. Coherent with these findings, RA proved to increase the proliferation of human fetal lung capillary endothelial precursor cells in a concentration-dependent manner, suggesting that RA ability to recover disrupted alveolarization is related to its direct influence in lung angiogenesis (Cho *et al.*, 2005). Regarding oxygen-induced lung injury, data indicates that newborn rats exposed to hyperoxia display impaired lung septation, decreased elastin content, larger mean lung volumes, larger alveoli, and decreased gas-exchange tissue relative to air-exposed animals (Randell *et al.*, 1989; Veness-Meehan *et al.*, 1994, 2000, 2002). Fourteen days after RA administration to these animals, survival rates and collagen deposition were increased, but septal formation and airspace size had not improved (Veness-Meehan *et al.*, 2000). However, at postnatal day 42, RA-treated animals show normal septal formation, which suggests that RA can act as an antioxidant, protecting the lungs from oxygen free radicals generated through direct oxygen exposure and from inflammatory cells (Veness-Meehan *et al.*, 2002), in a mechanism mediated trough cytochrome P4501A enzymes (Couroucli *et al.*, 2006). Despite of this, in the adult rat lung vitamin A supplementation at either therapeutic or excessive doses induces lipid peroxidation, protein carbonylation, and oxidation of protein thiol groups, as well as change in catalase and superoxide dismutase activity, altering lung's redox balance (Pasquali *et al.*, 2009). Nevertheless, these findings should be regarded with caution, since vitamin A and RA effects are dose-dependent and regulated in a spatiotemporal manner, and therefore the pro-oxidant effects of vitamin A registered in the adult rat lung may not be present in the developing lung. Pulmonary hypoplasia, secondary to the relatively common congenital diaphragmatic hernia (CDH) is the main cause of the high morbidity and mortality in infants bearing this malformation (Doyle & Lally, 2004; Ivascu & Hirschl, 2004; Grosche *et al.*, 2005). In the nitrofen-model of CDH, retinol lung storage is decreased due to nitrofen interference with its cellular uptake during lung morphogenesis, leading to pulmonary hypoplasia (Nakasawa *et al.*, 2007). Prenatal administration of vitamin A (Baptista *et al.*, 2005), as well as exogenous RA added to fetal lung explants (Montedonico et al., 2006; Montedonico *et al.*, 2008) attenuates lung hypoplasia in the nitrofen-model of CDH. This effect is achieved, at least, by two complementary mechanisms: the first includes RA up-regulation of genes that are pattern regulators of lung morphogenesis, such as *COUP-TFII*, *Gata 4*, and *FOG 2* (Friend of Gata2) (Doi *et al.*, 2009), and the second RA-enhancement of alveolar cell type I proliferation (Sugimoto *et al.*, 2008). Furthermore, antenatal vitamin A also decreases ventilation-induced lung injury (Lewis *et al.*, 2006).

In the developed countries vitamin A supplementation is a common practice that significantly contributed to the reduction of infant mortality as well as the incidence of xerophthalmia, respiratory infection, and morbidity from gastrointestinal disease (Humphrey *et al.*, 1996; Roy *et al.*, 1997; Haidar *et al.*, 2003). When this supplementation is given within the 48 hours after birth, it reduces infant mortality by nearly a quarter, with the greatest benefit for low weight birth infants (Rahmathullah *et al.*, 2003). Premature infants, especially those of extremely low birth weight (ELBW) are at high risk for mortality, BPD, retinopathy of prematurity, and long-term neurodevelopment impairment (Ambalavanan *et al.*, 2005). These infants are born with low body stores of vitamin A, and are at high risk of vitamin A deficiency, which increases the risk of BPD, and are often unable to tolerate oral supplementation (Mactier & Weaver, 2004). During the period of January 1996-July 1997, Tyson and colleagues (1999) conducted a multicenter, randomized trial to determine the effectiveness and safety of a higher dose of vitamin A (5000 IU) than used in previous trials in ELBW, given by intramuscular route three times for week during four weeks. This trial indicated that at 36 corrected weeks, ELBW had lower risk of BPD and reduced biochemical evidence of vitamin A deficiency. Vitamin A intramuscular supplementation also decreased death or oxygen dependency by 1 month of age in preterm infants (Mactier & Weaver, 2004). In another clinical trial with a larger follow-up period, vitamin A supplementation given largely to infants less than 1 kg resulted in a decrease in death and/or BPD without increasing mortality or neurodevelopment impairment at 18 to 22 months (Ambalavanan *et al.*, 2005). In complex diseases such as BPD, the improvements in outcome are expected to occur gradually, but the overall findings of these clinical trials point out to the benefits of vitamin A supplementation in ELBW, providing evidence that it would be reasonable to implement routine supplementation of this micronutrient to premature infants. However, care must be taken and further investigation is needed to identify the safest dosage regimen and route of administration.

Chapter X

Conclusion

During fetal and perinatal development a coordinated series of molecular and cellular events shape the pulmonary complex architectural pattern. Lung morphogenesis follows a rigid morphogenetic hierarchy that determines how, when and where the processes of branching morphogenesis, cellular proliferation and differentiation, vessel development and overall growth will occur. Data presented in this chapter shows that vitamin A and it active metabolite, retinoic acid, are involved in lung morphogenesis since the earliest stages as pattern regulators. Furthermore, the morphological and biochemical studies here presented lead towards the conclusion that a criterious administration of vitamin A, in well determined doses and once the critical period of retinoid-induced teratogenesis is over, is advantageous for the fetus. The administration of Vitamin A during gestation favors the expression of vascular endothelial growth factor (VEGF) and modulates enzymes and molecules responsible for tissue remodeling (MMPs and TIMPs) in a way that enhances the lung morphogenesis and histogenesis. It also modulates the whole alveolarization process by the anticipation of the appearance of elastic fibers at the level of the lung's respiratory portion, as well as enhances pulmonary and hepatic retinoids storage capacity during gestation and in the postnatal period. These results are promising and can make an important contribution towards future, appropriately designed, strategies for preventing the risks associated with premature labor and the treatment of bronchopulmonary dysplasia. However, upon interpreting such studies in animal models it is important to be aware of the possible confounding influences of phenomena such as the differences between lung development and vitamin A pharmacokinetics in rodents and humans.

References

Abman, S.H. (2007). Recent advances in the pathogenesis and treatment of persistent pulmonary hypertension of the newborn. *Neonatol.*, *91*, 283-290.

Abman, S. (2003). Vascular endothelial growth factor: Not only for vessels anymore. *Pediatr. Res.*, *53*, 1, 1.

Adamson, I.Y., & King, G.M. (1984). Sex-related differences in cellular composition and surfactant synthesis of developing fetal rat lungs. *Am. Rev. Respir Dis.* , *1*, 130-134.

Ambalavanan N, Tyson JE, Kennedy KA, Hansen NI, Vohr BR, Wright LL, Carlo WA & National Institute of Child Health and Human Development Neonatal Research Network (2005) Vitamin A supplementation for extremely low birth wieght infants: outcome at 18 to 22 months. *Pediatrics, 115*, 249-254.

Antipatis, C. Ashworth, C.J., Grant, G., Lea, R.G., Hay, S.M., & Rees, W.D. (1998). Effects of maternal vitamin A status on fetal heart and lung: Changes in expression of key developmental genes. *Am. J. Physiol.*, *275*, L1184-L1191.

Antipatis, C., Ashworth, C.J., Grant, G., Lea, R.G., Hay, S.M., Rees, W.D. (2000). Moderate maternal vitamin A deficiency affects perinatal organ growth and development in rats. *Br J Nutr.* *84*, 1, 125-132.

Arceci, R.J., King, A.A., & Simon, M.C. (1993). Mouse GATA-4: A retinoic acid-inducible GATA-binding transcription factor expressed in endodermally derived tissues and heart. *Mol. Cell Biol.*, *13*, 4, 2235-2246.

Atkinson, J.J., & Senior, R.M. (2003). Matrix metalloproteinase-9 in lung remodeling. *Am. J. Respir Cell Mol Biol.*, *28*, 1, 12-24.

Balmer, J.E., & Blomhoff, R. (2002). Gene expression regulation by retinoic acid. *J. Lipid Res.*, *43*, 1773-1808.

Baptista, M.J., Melo-Rocha, G., Pedrosa, C., Gonzaga, S., Teles, A., Estevão-Costa, J., Areias, J.C., Flake, A.W., Leite-Moreira, A.F., & Correia-Pinto, J. (2005) Antenatal vitamin A administration attenuates lung hypoplasia by interfering with early instead of late determinants of lung underdevelopment in congenital diaphragmatic hernia. *J Pediatr Surg. 40*, 4, 658-665.

Barón, M.A., Solano, L., Llovera, D., & Peña, E. (2003). Vitamin A status in pregnant adolescents of low socioeconomic income. *Arch. Latinoam Nutr. 53*,4, 364-368.

Bellusci, S., Grindley, J., Emoto, H., Itoh, N., & Hogan, B.L. (1997). Fibroblast growth factor 10 (FGF10) and branching morphogenesis in the embryonic mouse lung. *Development*, *124*, 4867-4878.

Bellusci, S., Grindley, J., Emoto, H., Itoh, N., & Hogan, B.L. (1997). Fibroblast growth factor 10 (FGF10) and branching morphogenesis in the embryonic mouse lung. *Development*, *124*, 4867-4878.

Bhatt, A.J., Pryhuber, G.S., Huyck, H., Watkins, R.H., Metlay, L.A., & Maniscalco, W.M. (2001). Disrupted pulmonary vasculature and decreased vascular endothelial growth factor, Flt-1, and TIE-2 in human infants dying with bronchopulmonary dysplasia. *Am. J. Respir Crit Care Med., 164*, 1971–1980.

Blomhoff, R., Green, M.H., Berg, T., & Norum, K. (1990). Transport and storage of vitamin A. *Science*, *250*, 399-404.

Bruce, M.C., & Honaker, C.E. (1998). Transcriptional regulation of tropoelastin expression in rat lung fibroblasts: Changes with age and hyperoxia. *Am. J. Physiol.*, *274*, L940-L950.

Burri, P.H. (2006). Structural aspects of postnatal lung development -Alveolar formation and growth. *Biol Neonate*, *89*, 313–322.

Burri, P.H. (1991). Postnatal development and growth. In: R.G. Crystal, J.B. West,P.J. Barnes,N.S. Cherniack, & E.R. Weibel, (eds.). *The Lung: Scientific Foundations*. New York: Raven Press, pp. 677-687.

Burri, PH. (1974). The postnatal growth of the rat lung: 3 Morphology. *Anat. Rec. 180*, 77-98.

Cardoso, W.V. (2001). Molecular regulation of lung development. *Ann .Rev. Physiol.*, *63*, 471-494.

Cardoso, W.V. (2004). Lung morphogenesis, role of growth factors and transcription factors In: R. Harding, K.E. Pinkerton, & C.G. Plopper, (eds.) *The Lung-Development, Aging and the Environment*. London: Elsevier,pp. 8-9.

Cardoso, W.V., & Lü, J. (2006). Regulation of early lung morphogenesis: Questions, facts and controversies. *Development*, *133*, 1611-1624.

Cardoso, W.V., Mitsialis, S.A., Brody, J.S., & Williams, M.C. (1996). Retinoic acid alters the expression of pattern-related genes in the developing rat lung. *Dev. Dyn.* *207*, 1, 47-59.

Cardoso, W.V., Williams, M.C., Mitsialis, S.A., Joyce-Brady, M., Rishi, A.K., & Brody, J.S. (1995). Retinoic acid induces changes in the pattern of airway branching and alters epithelial cell differentiation in the developing lung *in vitro*. *Am. J. Respir. Cell Mol Biol.* *12*, *5*, 464-476.

Carey, M.A., Card, J.W., Voltz, J.W., Arbes, S.J., Jr., Germolec, D.R., Korach, K.S., & Zeldin, D.C. (2007). It's all about sex: Gender, lung development and lung disease. *Trends Endocrinol Metab.* *18*, 8, 308-313.

Chailley-Heu, B., Chelly, N., Lelièvre-Pégorier, M., Barlier-Mur, A.M., Merlet-Bénichou, C., & Bourbon, J.R. (1999). Mild vitamin A deficiency delays fetal lung maturation in the rat. *Am. J. Respir. Cell Mol. Biol.* *21*, 1, 89-96.

Chakrabarti, S., & Patel, K.D. (2005). Matrix metalloproteinase-2 (MMP-2) and MMP-9 in pulmonary pathology. *Exp. Lung Res.*, *31*, 6, 599-621.

Chazaud, C., Chambon, P., & Dollé, P. (1999). Retinoic acid is required in the mouse embryo for left-right asymmetry determination and heart morphogenesis. *Development*, *126*, 12, 2589-2596.

Chen, F., Desai, T.J., Qian, J., Niederreither, K., Lu, J., & Cardoso, W.V. (2007). Inhibition of Tgf beta signaling by endogenous retinoic acid is essential for primary lung bud induction. *Development*, *134*, 2969-2979.

Cho, S.J., George, C.L.S., Snyder. J.M-. Acarregui. M.J-(2005) Retinoic acid and erythropoietin maintain alveolar development in mice treated with an angiogenesis inhibitor. *Am. J. Respir. Cell. Mol. Biol.*, 33:622–628.

Chytil, F. (1992). The lungs and vitamin A. *Am. J. Physiol.*, *262*, L517-L527.

Couroucli, X.I., Liang, Y.W., Jiang, W., Barrios, R., & Moorthy, B. (2006). Attenuation of oxygen-induced abnormal lung maturation in rats by retinoic acid: Possible role of cytochrome P4501A enzymes. *J. Pharmacol. Exp. Ther.*, *317*, 3, 946-954.

Croskerry, P.G., Smith G.K., Hall, S., Shepard, B.J.. (1978) Fetal and placental growth in the rat following differential reduction of litter size.. *Biol Neonate*, *33*, 31-38..

De Moerlooze, L., Spencer-Dene, B., Revest, J., Hajihosseini, M., Rosewell, I., Dickson, C. (2000). An important role for the IIIb isoform of fibroblast growth factor receptor 2 (FGFR2) in mesenchymal-epithelial signaling during mouse organogenesis. *Development*, *127*, 483-492.

Del Moral, P., Sala, F.G., Tefft, D., Shi, W., Keshet, E., Bellusci, S., Warburton, D. (2006). VEGF-A signaling through Flk-1 is a critical facilitator of early embryonic lung epithelial to endothelial crosstalk and branching morphogenesis. *Dev. Biol.*, *290*, 177-188.

De Luca, L.M., & McDowell, L.M. (1989). Effects of vitamin A status on hamster tracheal epithelium in vivo and vitro. *Food Nutr.Bull.*, *11*, 20-24.

Desai, T.J., Chen, F., Lu, J., Qian, J., Niederreither, K., Dollé, P. Chambon, P., & Cardoso, W.V. (2006). Distinct roles for retinoic acid receptors alpha and beta in early lung morphogenesis. *Dev. Biol.*, *291*, 12-24.

Desai, T.J., Malpel, S., Flentke, G.R., Smith, S.M., & Cardoso, W.V. (2004). Retinoic acid selectively regulates Fgf10 expression and maintains cell identity in the prospective lung field of the developing foregut. *Dev. Biol.*, *273*, 402-415.

Dirami, G., Massaro, G.D., Clerch, L.B., Ryan, U.S., Reczek, P.R., Massaro, D. (2004). Lung retinol storing cells synthesize and secrete retinoic acid, an inducer of alveolus formation. *Am J Physiol. Lung Cell Mol. Physiol.*, *286*, 2, L249-L256.

Doi, T., Sugimoto, K., & Puri, P. (2009). Prenatal retinoic acid up-regulates pulmonary gene expression of COUP-TFII, FOG2, and GATA4 in pulmonary hypoplasia. *J. Pediatr. Surg.* *44*, 10, 1933-1937.

Dollé, P. (2009). Developmental expression of retinoic acid receptors (RARs). *Nucl. Recept. Signal.*, *12*,7,e006.

Dollé, P., Ruberte, E., Leroy, P., Morriss-Kay, G., & Chambon, P. (1990). Retinoic acid receptors and retinoic acid binding proteins. I. A systematic study of their differential pattern of transcription during mouse organogenesis. *Development*, *110*,1133-1151.

Doyle, N.M., & Lally, K.P. (2004). The CDH Study Group and advance in the clinical care of the patient with congenital diaphragmatic hernia. *Semin. Perinatol.*, *28*,174-184.

Fleisher, B., Kulovich, M.V., Hallman, M. & Gluck, L. (1985). Lung profile: Sex differences in normal pregnancy. *Obstet. Gynecol.*, *66*, 3, 327-330.

Fujita, M., Ye, Q., Ouchi, H., Nakashima, N., Hamada, N., Hagimoto, N., Kuwano, K., Mason, R.J., & Nakanishi, Y. (2004). Retinoic acid fails to reverse emphysema in adult mouse models. *Thorax* *59*, 224-230.

Fukuda, Y., Ferrans, V.J., & Crystal, R.G. (1984). Development of elastic fibers of nuchal ligament, aorta, and lung of fetal and postnatal sheep: An ultrastructural and electron microscopic immunohistochemical study. *Am. J. Anat., 170*, 597-629.

Geevarghese, S.K., & Chytil, F. (1994). Depletion of retinyl esters in the lungs coincides with lung prenatal morphological maturation. *Biochem. Biophys. Res. Commun., 200*, 529-535.

Gray, T., Koo, J.S., & Nettesheim, P. (2001). Regulation of mucous differentiation and mucin gene expression in the tracheobronchial epithelium. *Toxicology, 160*, 35-46.

Greenlee, K.J., Werb, Z., & Kheradmand, F. (2007). Matrix metalloproteinases in lung: Multiple, multifarious, and multifaceted. *Physiol. Rev. 87*, 1, 69-98.

Grosche, J.R., Islam, S., &Boulanger, S.C. (2005). Congenital diaphragmatic hernia. *Am. J. Surg., 190*, 324-332.

Gueders, M.M., Foidart, J.M., Noel, A., & Cataldo, D.D. (2006). Matrix metalloproteinases (MMPs) and tissue inhibitors of MMPs in the respiratory tract: Potential implications in asthma and other lung diseases. *Eur. J. Pharmacol. 533*, 1-3;133-144.

Haidar, J., Tsegaye, D., Maiam, D.H., Tibeb, H.N., & Muroki, N.M. (2003). Vitamin A supplementation on child morbidity. *E Afr. Med. J. 80*, 17-21.

Healy, A.M., Margenthau, L., Zhu, X., Farber, H.W., & Cardoso, W.V. (2000). VEGF is deposited in the subepithelial matrix at the leading edge of branching airways and stimulates neovascularization in the murine embryonic lung. *Dev. Dyn., 219*, 341-352.

Heine, U. I., Munoz, E.F., Flanders, K.C., Roberts, A.B., & Sporn, M.B. (1990) Colocalization of TGF-beta 1 and collagen I and III, fibronectin and glycosaminoglycans during lung branching morphogenesis. *Development, 109*, 29-36.

Hind, M., & Maden, M. (2004). Retinoic acid induces alveolar regeneration in the adult mouse lung. Retinoic acid induces alveolar regeneration in the adult mouse lung. *Eur. Respir. J., 23*, 20-27.

Hislop, A.A. (2002). Airway and blood vessel interaction during lung development. *J. Anat., 201*, 325-34.

Humphrey, J.H., Agoestina, T., Wu, L., Usman, A., Nurachim, M., Subardja, D., Hidayat, S., Tielsch, J., West, K.P., Jr., & Sommer, (1996). Impact of neonatal vitamin A supplementation on infant morbidity and mortality. *J. Pediatr. 128*, 489-496.

Hustead, V.A., Gutcher, G.R., Anderson, S.A., & Zachman, R.D.(1984). Relationship of vitamin A (retinol) status to lung disease in the pre-term infant. *J. Pediatr., 105*, 610-611.

Inder, T.E., Graham, P.J., Winterbourn, C.C., Austin, N.C., & Darlow, B.A. (1998). Plasma vitamin A levels in the very low birthweight infant: Relationship to respiratory outcome. *Early Hum. Dev., 52*, 155-168.

Ivascu, F.A., & Hirschl, R.B. (2004). New approaches to managing congenital diaphragmatic hernia. *Semin Perinatol., 28*,185-198.

Jakkula, M., Le Cras, T.D., Gebb, S., Hirth, K.P., Tuder, R.M., Voelkel, N.F., Abman, S.H. (2000). Inhibition of angiogenesis decreases alveolarization in the developing rat lung. *Am. J. Physiol Lung Cell Mol. Physiol., 279*, 3, L600-L607.

Jeffery, P.K. (1998). The development of large and small airways. *Am. J. Respir. Crit. Care Med., 157*, S174-S180.

Joshi, S., & Kotecha, S. (2007). Lung growth and development. *Early Hum. Dev., 83*, 789-794.

Kaner, R.J., & Crystal, R.G. (2001). Compartmentalization of vascular endothelial growth factor to the epithelial surface of the human lung. *Mol. Med. 7*, 240-246.

Kaner, R.J., Ladetto, J.V., Singh, R., Fukuda, N., Matthay, M.A., & Crystal, R.G. (2000). Lung overexpression of the vascular endothelial growth factor gene induces pulmonary edema. *Am. J. Respir Cell Mol. Biol., 22*, 657-664.

Kotesha, S. (2000).Lung growth for beginners. *Paediatr Respir Rev., 1*, 4, 308-313.

Kumar, V.H., Lakshminrusimha, S., Abiad, M.T., Chess, P.R., & Ryan, R.M. (2005). Growth factors in lung development. *Adv. Clin. Chem., 40*, 261-316.

Lai, L., Bohnsack, B.L., Niederreither, K., & Hirschi, K.K. (2003). Retinoic acid regulates endothelial cell proliferation during vasculogenesis. *Development, 130*, 6465-6474.

Lewis, N.A., Holm, A.B., Swartz, D., Sokolowski, J., Rossman, J., & Glick, P.L. (2006). Antenatal vitamin a decreases ventilation-induced lung injury in the lamb model of congenital diaphragmatic hernia. *Asian J. Surg., 29*, 3,193-197.

Lowe, L.A., Yamada, S., & Kuehn, M.R. (2001). Genetic dissection of nodal function in patterning the mouse embryo. *Development, 128*, 1831-1843.

Lucey, E.C., Goldstein, R.H., Breuer, R., Rexer, B.N., Ong, D.E., & Snider, G.L. (2003). Retinoic acid does not affect alveolar septation in adult FVB mice with elastase-induced emphysema. *Respiration, 70*, 200-205.

Ludwig, M.G., Basset, P., & Anglard, P. (2000). Multiple regulatory elements in the murine stromelysin-3 promoter. Evidence for direct control by

CCAAT/enhancer-binding protein b and thyroid and retinoid receptors. *J. Biol. Chem.*, *275*, 39981-39990.

Mactier, H., & Weaver, L.T. (2005).Viatamin A and pre-term infants: What we know, what we don't know, and what we need to know. *Arch Dis Child Fetal Neonatal.*, *90*, F103-108.

Maden, M. (2006). Retinoids have different efficacies on alveolar regeneration in a dexamethasone-treated mouse. *Am. J. Respir. Cell Mol .Biol.*, *35*, 260-267.

Maden, M., & Hind, M. (2004). Retinoic acid in alveolar development, maintenance and regeneration. *Phil Trans R Soc. Lond.*, B, *359*, 799-808.

Malpel, S., Mendelsohn, C., & Cardoso, W.V. (2000). Regulation of retinoic acid signaling during lung morphogenesis. *Development*, *127*, 3057-3067

March, T.H., Bowen, L.E., Finch, G.L., Nikula, K.J., Wayne, B.J., & Hobbs, C.H. (2005). Effects of strain and treatment with inhaled aIl-trans-retinoic acid on cigarette smoke-induced pulmonary emphysema in mice. *COPD, 2*, 289-302.

March, T.H., Cossey, P.Y., Esparza, D.C., Dix, K.J., McDonald, J.D., & Bowen, L.E. (2004). Inhalation administration of all-trans-retinoic acid for treatment of elastase-induced pulmonary emphysema in Fischer 344 rats. *Exp. Lung Res.*, *30*, 383-404.

Mark, M., Ghyselinck, N.B., & Chambon, P. (2006). Function of retinoid nuclear receptors: Lessons from genetic and pharmacological dissections of the retinoic acid signaling pathway during mouse embryogenesis. *Ann. Rev. Pharmacol Toxicol.*, *46*, 451-480.

Massaro, D., & Massaro, G. (2006). Estrogen receptor regulation of pulmonary alveolar dimensions: Alveolar sexual dimorphism in mice. *Am. J. Physiol Lung Cell Mol. Physiol.*, *290*, L866-L870.

Massaro, D., & Massaro, G. (2004). Estrogen regulates pulmonary alveolar formation, loss, and regeneration in mice. *Am. J. Physiol Lung Cell Mol. Physiol.*, *287*, L1154-L1159.

Massaro, G.D., & Massaro, D. (1997). Retinoic acid treatment abrogates elastase-induced pulmonary emphysema in rats. *Nat Med. 6*, 675-677.

Massaro, G.D., Massaro, D., Chan, W.Y., Clerch, L.B., Ghyselinck, N., Chambon, P., & Chandraratna, R.A. (2000). Retinoic acid receptor-beta: An endogenous inhibitor of the perinatal formation of pulmonary alveoli. *Physiol. Genomics*, *4*, 51-57.

Massaro, G.M., Mortola, J.P., & Massaro, D. (1996). Estrogen modulates the dimensions of the lung's gas-exchange surface area and alveoli in female rats. *Am. J. Physiol Lung Cell Mol. Physiol.*, *270*, L110-L114.

Massaro, G.M., Mortola, J.P., & Massaro, D. (1995). Sexual dimorphism in the architecture of the lung's gas-exchange region. *PNAS*, *92*, 1105-1107.

Mauroy, B., Filoche, M., Weibel, E.R., & Sapoval, B. (2004). An optimal bronchial tree may be dangerous. *Nature*, *427*, 633-636.

McDowell, E.M., Ben, T., Coleman, B., Chang, S., Newkirk, C., & De Luca, L.M. (1987). Effects of retinoic acid on the growth and morphology of hamster tracheal epithelial cells in primary culture. *Virchows Arch B Cell Pathol Incl. Mol. Pathol.*, *54*, 1, 38-51.

McGowan, S., Jackson, S.K., Jenkins-Moore, M., Dai, H.H., Chambon, P., & Snyder, J.M. (2000). Mice bearing deletions of retinoic acid receptors demonstrate reduced lung elastin and alveolar numbers. *Am. J. Respir Cell Mol. Biol.*, *23*, 162-167.

McGowan, S.E., Doro, M.M., & Jackson, S.K. (1997). Endogenous retinoids increase perinatal elastin gene expression in rat lung fibroblasts and fetal explants. *Am. J. Physiol.*, *273*, L410-L416.

McGowan, S.E., Harvey, C.S., & Jackson, S.K. (1995). Retinoids, retinoic acid receptors, and cytoplasmic retinoid binding proteins in perinatal rat lung fibroblasts. *Am. J. Physiol Lung Cell Mol Physiol.*, *269*, L463-L472.

McGowan, S.E., & Snyder, J.M. (2004). Development of alveoli. In: R. Harding, K.E. Pinkerton, & C.G. Plopper, (eds.) *The Lung-Development, Aging and the Environment.* London: Elsevier,pp. 55-68.

McKeown, T., Marshall, T., & Record, R.G. (1976). Influences on fetal growth. *J. Reprod Fertil.*, *47*, 1, 167-181.

McMillan, E.M., King, G.M., & Adamson, I.Y. (1989). Sex hormones influence growth and surfactant production in fetal lung explants. *Exp Lung Res.* *15*, 2, 167-179.

Mendelsohn, C., Lohnes, D., Décimo, D., Lufkin, T., LeMeur, M., Chambon, P., & Mark, M. (1994). Function of the retinoic acid receptors (RARs) during development. II. Multiple abnormalities at various stages of organogenesis in RAR double mutants. *Development*, *120*, 2749-2771.

Mollard, R., Viville, S., Ward, S.J., Décimo, D., Chambon, P., & Dollé, P. (2000). Tissue-specific expression of retinoic acid isoform transcripts in the mouse embryo. *Mech. Dev.*, *94*, 223-232.

Montedonico, S., Nakazawa, N., & Puri, P. (2006). Retinoic acid rescues lung hypoplasia in nitrofen-induced hypoplastic foetal rat lung explants. *Pediatr. Surg Int.*, *22*, 1, 2-8.

Montedonico, S., Sugimoto, K., Felle, P., Bannigan, J., & Puri, P. (2008). Prenatal treatment with retinoic acid promotes pulmonary alveologenesis in the nitrofen model of congenital diaphragmatic hernia. *J. Pediatr Surg. 43*, 3, 500-507.

Morabia, A., Menkes, M.J., Comstock, G.W., & Tockman, M.S. (1990). Serum retinol and airway obstruction. *Am J Epidemiol., 132*, 77-82.

Nakazawa, N., Montedonico, S., Takayasu, H., Paradisi, F., & Puri, P. (2007). Disturbance of retinol transportation causes nitrofen-induced hypoplastic lung. *J. Pediatr. Surg. 42*, 2, 345-349.

Ngare, D.K., Muttunga, J.N., & Njonge, E. (2000). Vitamin A deficiency in pre-school children in Kenya. *East Afr. Med. J. 77*, 8, 421-424.

Okabe, T., Yorifuji, H., Yamada, E., & Takaku, F. (1984). Isolation and characterization of vitamin-A-storing lung cells. *Exp. Cell Res., 154*, 1, 125-135.

Parera, M.C., van Dooren, M., van Kempen, A., Krijger, D., Grosveld, F., Tiboel, D., & Rottier, R. (2005). Distal angiogenesis: A new concept for lung vascular morphogenesis. *Am. J. Physiol. Lung Cell Mol. Physiol., 288*:L141-L149.

Park, W.Y., Miranda, B., Lebeche, D., Hashimoto, G., & Cardoso, W.V.(1998). FGF-10 is achemotactic factor for distal epithelial buds during lung development. *Dev. Biol., 201*, 125-134.

Pasquali, M.A., Gelain, D.P., de Oliveira, M.R., Behr, G.A., da Motta, L.L., da Rocha, R.F., Klamt, F., & Moreira, J.C. (2009). Vitamin A supplementation for different periods alters oxidative parameters in lungs of rats. *J. Med. Food. 12*, 6, 1375-1380.

Pierce, R.A., Joyce, B., Officer, S., Heintz, C., Moore, C., McCurnin, D., Johnston, C., & Maniscalco, W. (2007). Retinoids increase lung elastin expression but fail to alter morphology or angiogenesis genes in premature ventilated baboons. *Pediatr. Res. 61*, 6, 703-709.

Pinto, M.de L., Rodrigues, P., Coelho, A.C., Pires, M. dos A., dos Santos, D.L., Gonçalves, C., & Bairos, V.A. (2007). Prenatal administration of vitamin A alters pulmonary and plasma levels of vascular endothelial growth factor in the developing mouse. *Int. J. Exp. Pathol., 88*, 6, 393-401.

Plopper, C.G., & Fanucchi, M.V. (2004) Development of airway epithelium. In: R. Harding, K.E. Pinkerton, & C.G. Plopper, (eds.) *The Lung-Development, Aging and the Environment*. London: Elsevier, pp. 13-32.

Rahmathullah, L., Tielsch, J.M., Thulasiraj, R.D., Katz, J., Coles, C., Devi, S., John, R., Prakash, K., Sadanand, A.V., Edwin, N., & Kamaraj, C. (2003). Impact of supplementing newborn infants with vitamin A on early infant mortality: Community based randomized trial in southern India. *Brit. Med. J. 327*, 254-257.

Randell, S.H., Mercer, R.R., & Young, S.L. (1989). Postnatal growth of pulmonary acini and alveoli in normal and oxygen-exposed rats studied by serial section reconstructions response to vitamin A administration in infants susceptible to bronchopulmonary dysplasia. *J. Pediatr., 116*, 607-614.

Rodrigues, P., Gonçalves, C. & Bairos, V, (2004) Metabolic pathways and modulating effects of vitamin A. *Curr. Med. Chem. Immun. Endoc. Metab. Agents, 4*, 119-142.

Roy, S.K., Islam, A., Molla, A., Akramuzzaman, S.M., Jahan, F., & Fuchs, G. (1997). Impact of a single megadose of vitamin A at delivery on breastmilk of mothers and morbidity of their infants. *Eur. J. Clin. Nutr., 51*, 302-307.

Schellenberg, J.C., Liggins, G.C., & Stewart, A.W. (1987) Growth, elastin concentration, and collagen concentration of perinatal rat lung: effects of dexamethasone. *Pediatr. Res., 21,* 603-607.

Sekine, K., Ohuchi, H., Fujiwara, M., Yamasaki, M., Yoshizawa, T., Sato, T., Yagishita, N., Matsui, D., Koga, Y., & Itoh, N. (1999). Fgf10 is essential for limb and lung formation. *Nat. Genet., 21*, 138-141.

Serra, R., & Moses, H.L. (1995) pRb is necessary for inhibition of N-myc expression by TGF-beta 1 in embryonic lung organ cultures. *Development, 121*, 3057-3066.

Shenai, J.P., & Chytil, F. (1990). Vitamin A storage in lungs during perinatal development in the rat. *Biol. Neonate, 57*, 2, 126-132.

Shenai, J.P., Rush, M.G., Stahlman, M.T., & Chytil, F. (1990). Plasma retinol-binding protein response to vitamin A administration in infants susceptible to bronchopulmonary dysplasia.. *J. Pediatr., 116*, 4, 607-614.

Shi, W., Chen,F., & Cardoso, W.V. (2009). Mechanisms of Lung Development. Contribution to Adult Lung Disease and Relevance to Chronic Obstructive Pulmonary Disease. *The Proceedings of the American Thoracic Society 6*, 558-563.

Shinkai, M., Shinkai, T., Montedonico, S., & Puri, P. (2006). Effect of VEGF on the branching morphogenesis of normal and nitrofen-induced hypoplastic fetal rat lung explants. *J. Ped. Surg., 41*, 781-786.

Sommer, A. (2003). Vitamin A deficiency and the global response. *Forum. Nutr. 56*, 33-35.

Spit, B.J. (1983). Induction of lipid droplets in fibroblasts of the hamster lung by a diet high in vitamin A. *Exp. Lung Res., 4*, 4, 247-257.

Srinivasan, G., Bruce, E.N., Houtz, P.K., & Bruce, M.C. (2002). Dexamethasone- induced changes in lung function are not prevented by concomitant treatment with retinoic acid. *Am J Physiol Lung Cell Mol. Physiol., 283*, L275-L287.

Stenmark, K.R., & Abman, S.H. (2005). Lung vascular development: Implications for the pathogenesis of bronchopulmonary dysplasia. *Ann. Rev. Physiol., 67*,623-661.

Sugimoto, K., Takayasu, H., Nakazawa, N., Montedonico, S., & Puri, P. (2008). Prenatal treatment with retinoic acid accelerates type 1 alveolar cell proliferation of the hypoplastic lung in the nitrofen model of congenital diaphragmatic hernia. *J. Pediatr. Surg. 43*, 2, 367-372.

Tepper, J., Pfeiffer, J., Aldrich, M., Tumas, D., Kern, J., Hoffman, E., McLennan, G., & Hyde, D. (2000). Can retinoic acid ameliorate the physiologic and morphologic effects of elastase instillation in the rat? *Chest, 117*,5, 242S-244S.

Thébaud, B., & Abman, S.H. (2007). Bronchopulmonary dysplasia: Where have all the vessels gone? Roles of angiogenic growth factors in chronic lung disease. *Am. J. Respir Crit. Care Med. 175*, 10, 978-985.

Thomas, M.R., Marston, L., Rafferty, G.F., Calvert, S., Marlow, N., Peacock, J.L., & Greenough, A. (2006). Respiratory function of very prematurely born infants at follow up: Influence of sex. *Arch. Dis. Child Fetal Neonatal Ed, 91*, 3, 197-201.

Torday, J., Hua, J., & Slavin, R. (1995). Metabolism and fate of neutral lipids of fetal lung fibroblast origin. *Biochim Biophys Acta., 1254*, 198-206.

Torday, J.S. (1984). The sex difference in type II cell surfactant synthesis originates in the fibroblast *in vitro*. *Exp. Lung Res. 7*, 187-194.

Torday, J.S., & Rehan, V.K. (2004). Does "A" stand for alveolization? *Eur. Respir. J., 23*,3-4.

Trotter, A., Kipp, M., Schrader, R.M., & Beyer, C. (2009a). Combined application of 17beta-estradiol and progesterone enhance vascular endothelial growth factor and surfactant protein expression in cultured embryonic lung cells of mice. *Int J Pediatr., 2009*, 170491

Trotter, A., Hilgendorff, A., Kipp, M., Beyer, C., Kueppers, E., Kiossis. E., Stuplich. J., Pohlandt, F., & Thome , U. (2009b) Gender-related effects of prenatal administration of estrogen and progesterone receptor antagonists on VEGF and surfactant-proteins and on alveolarisation in the developing piglet lung. *Early Hum. Dev., 85*, 6, 353-359

Tyson, J.E., Wright, L.L., Oh, W., Kennedy, K.A., Mele, L., Ehrenkranz, R.A., Stoll, B.J., Lemons, J.A., Stenvenson, D.K., Bauer, C.R., Korones,

S.B., & Fanaroff, A. (1999). Vitamin A supplementation for extremely-low-birth-weight infants. *N.Engl. J. Med.*, *340*,1962-1968.

Veness-Meehan, K.A., Bottone, F.G.. Jr., & Stiles, A.D. (2000). Effects of retinoic acid on airspace development and lung collagen in hyperoxia-exposed newborn rats. *Pediatr. Res.* *48*, 4, 434-444.

Veness-Meehan, K.A., Pierce, R.A., Moats-Staats, B.M., & Stiles, A.D. (2002). Retinoic acid attenuates O2-induced inhibition of lung septation. *Am. J. Physiol Lung Cell Mol. Physiol.* *283*, 5, L971-L980.

Veness-Meehan, K.A., Rhodes, D.N., & Stiles, A.D. (1994). Temporal and spatial expression of biglycan in chronic oxygen-induced lung injury. *Am. J. Resp Cell Mol. Biol.*, *11*, 509-524.

Verma, R.P., McCulloch, K.M., Worrell, L., & Vidyasagar, D. (1996). Vitamin A deficiency and severe bronchopulmonary dysplasia in very low birth weight infants. *Am. J. Perinatol.*, *13*, 389-393.

Voelkel, N.F., Vandivier, R.W., & Tuder, R.M. (2006). Vascular endothelial growth factor in the lung. *Am J. Physiol Lung Cell Mol. Physiol.*, *290*, L209-L221.

Wang, Z., Dollé, P., Cardoso, W.V., & Niederreither, K. (2006). Retinoic acid regulates morphogenesis and patterning of posterior foregut derivatives. *Dev. Biol.*, *297*, 433-445.

Warburton, D., Schwarz. M., Tefft, D., Flores-Delgado, G., Anderson, K.D., & Cardoso, W.V. (2000) The molecular basis of lung morphogenesis. *Mech. Dev.*, *92*, 55-81.

Wei, H., Huang, H-M., Li, T-Y., Qu, P., Liu, Y-X., & Chen, J. (2009). Marginal vitamin A deficiency affects lung maturation in rats from prenatal to adult stage. *J. Nutr. Sci. Vitaminol.*, *55*, 208-214.

Wert, S.E., Glasser, S.W., Korfhagen, T.R., & Whitsett, J.A. (1993). Transcriptional elements from the human SP-C gene direct expression in the primordial respiratory epithelium of transgenic mice. *Dev. Biol.*, *156*, 2, 426-443.

Winkler, M. K., Foldes J K., Bunn R C. & Fowlkes J L. (2003) Implications for matrix metalloproteinases as modulators of pediatric lung disease. *Am. J. Physiol. Lung Cell. Mol. Physiol.*, *284*: L557-L565.

Wolbach, S., & Howe, P (1925) Tissue changes following deprivation of fat soluble A vitamin. *J. Exp. Med.*, *42*, 753–777.

Zachman, R.D., Samuels, D.P., Brand, J.M., Winston, J.F., & Pi, J.T. (1996). Use of the intramuscular relative-dose-response test to predict bronchopulmonary dysplasia in premature infants. *Am. J. Clin. Nutr.*, *63*, 123-153.

Index

D

E

F

G

H

I

K

L

M

N

O

P

R

S

T

V

X

Y